THE STORY OF CANCER
Volume 2

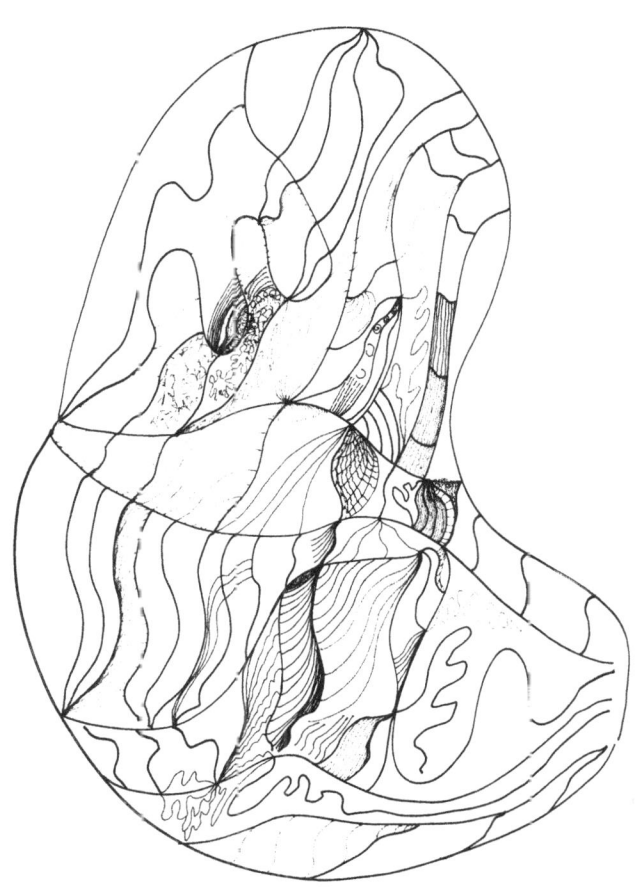

Camilia MacPherson, Ph.D., D.Th.
2016

INTRODUCTION

This is a continuation of one document with 7 volumes beginning with Volume 1.

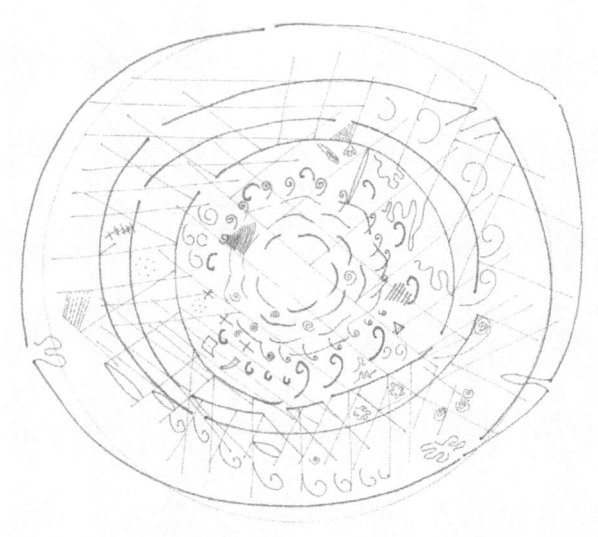

ISBN-13: 978-530542550
ISBN-10: 1530542553
Email: tamaracpublishers@icloud.com

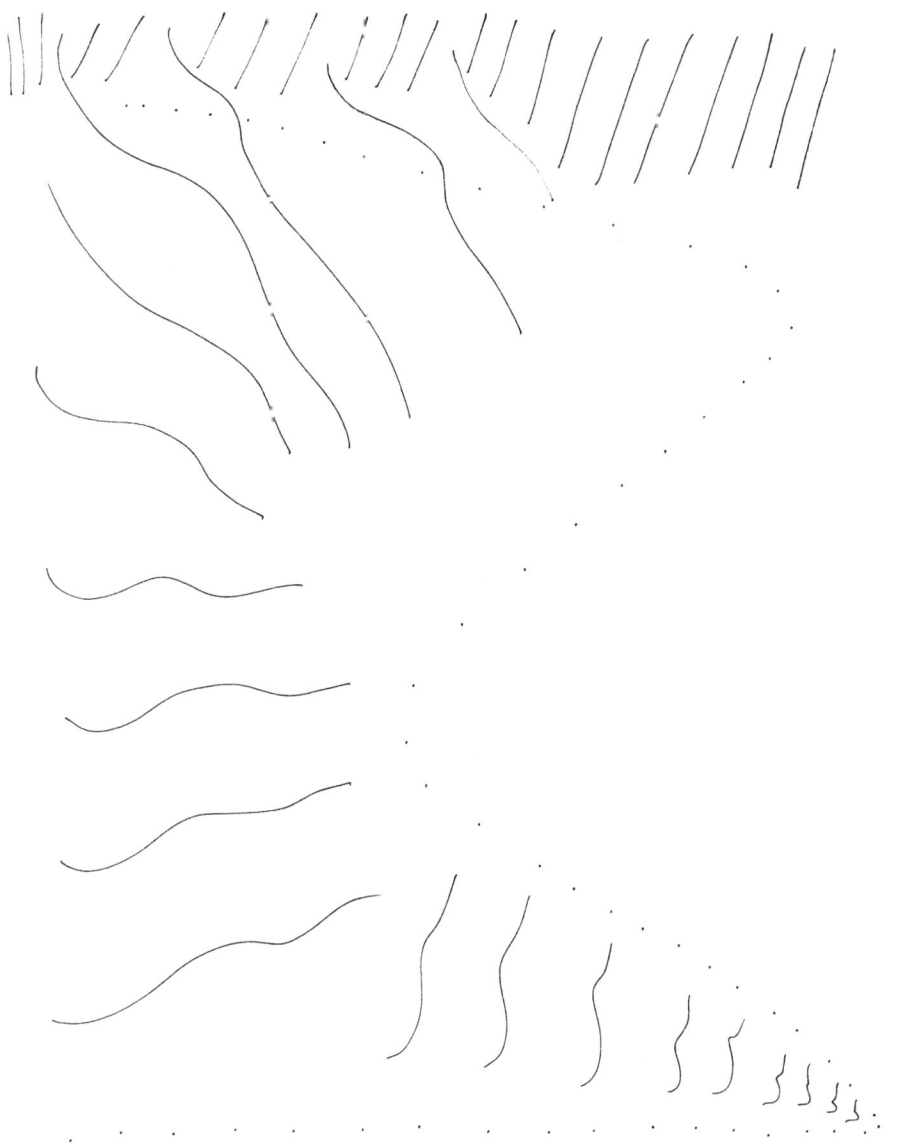

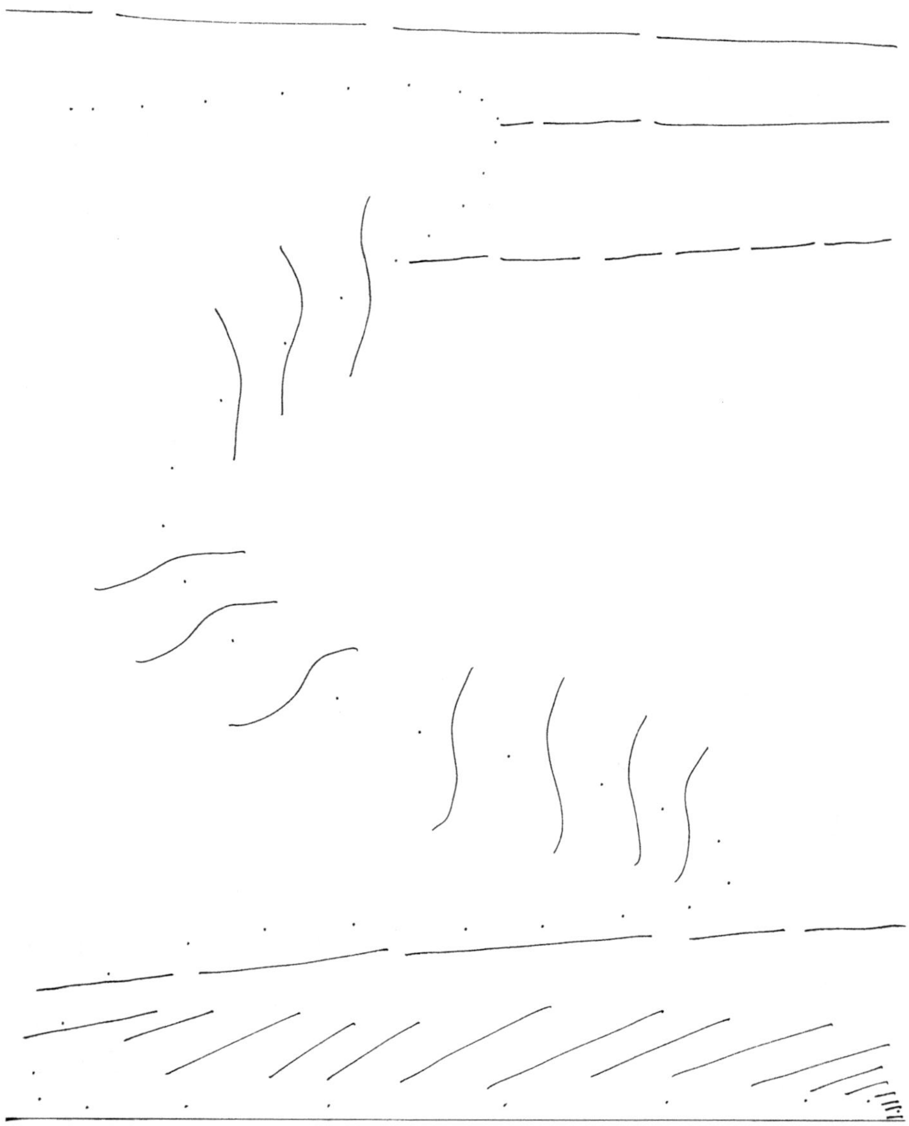

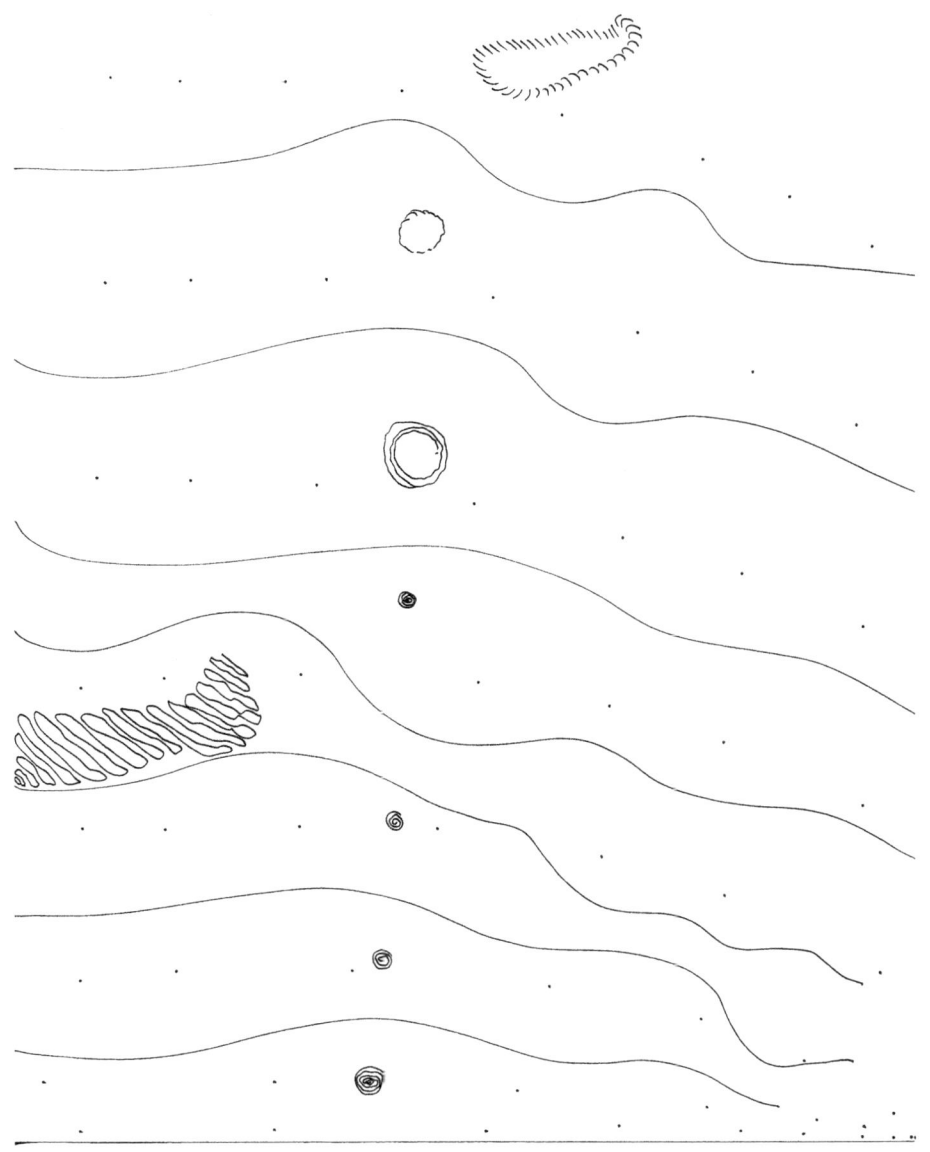

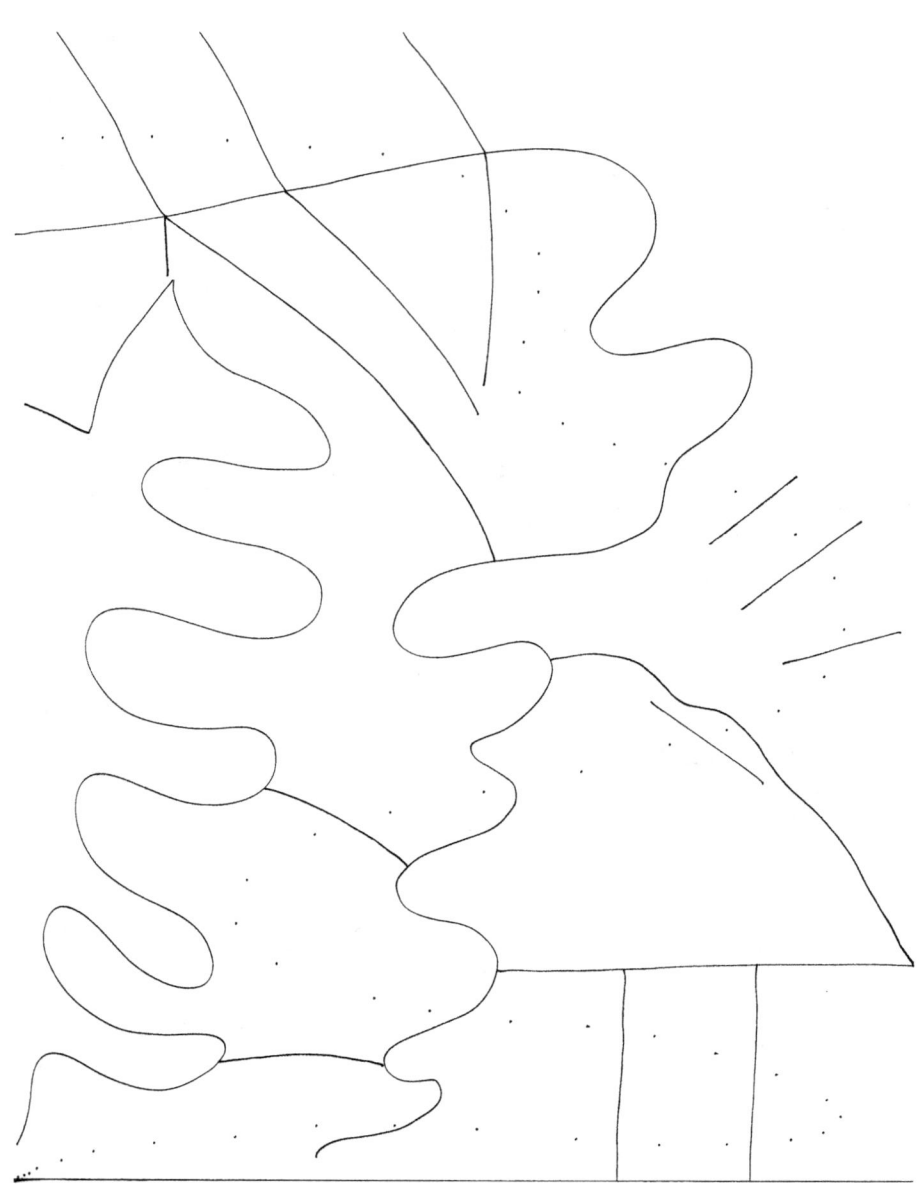

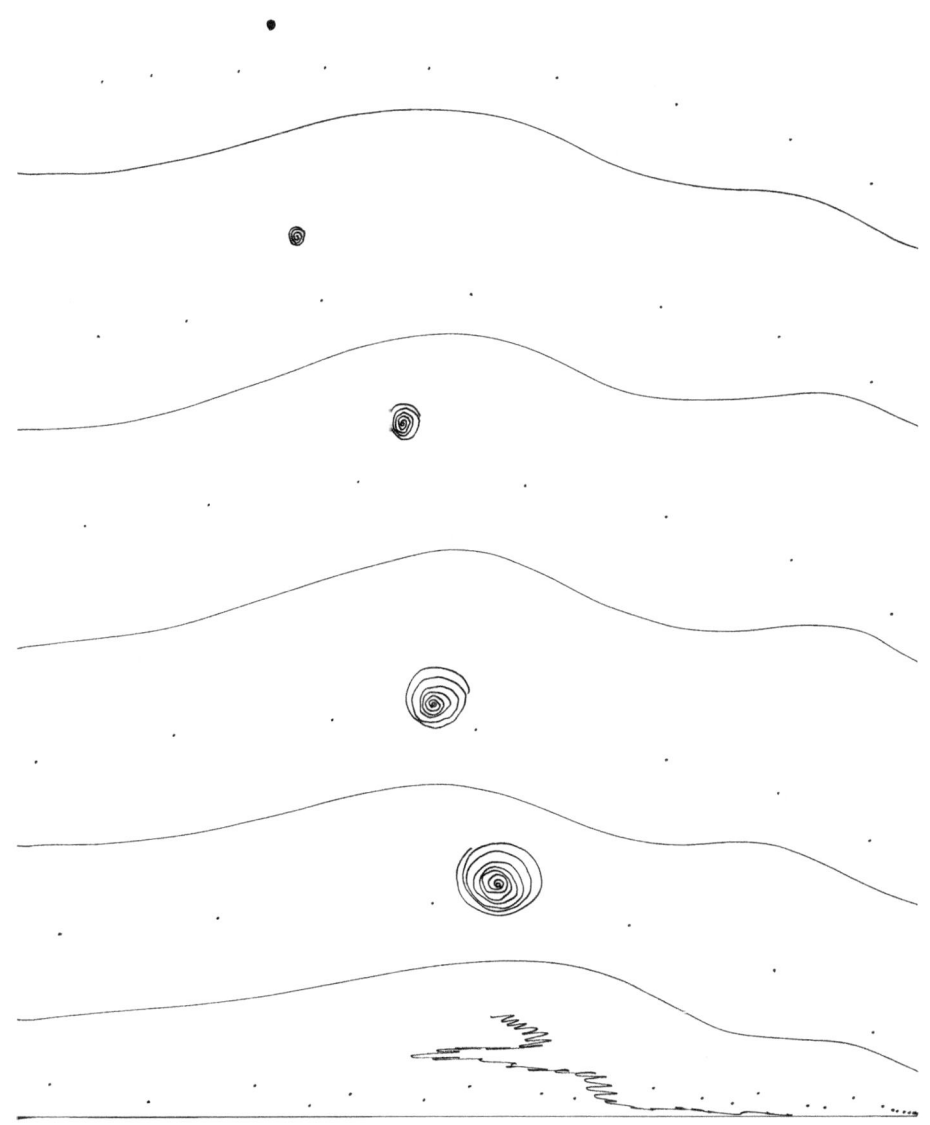

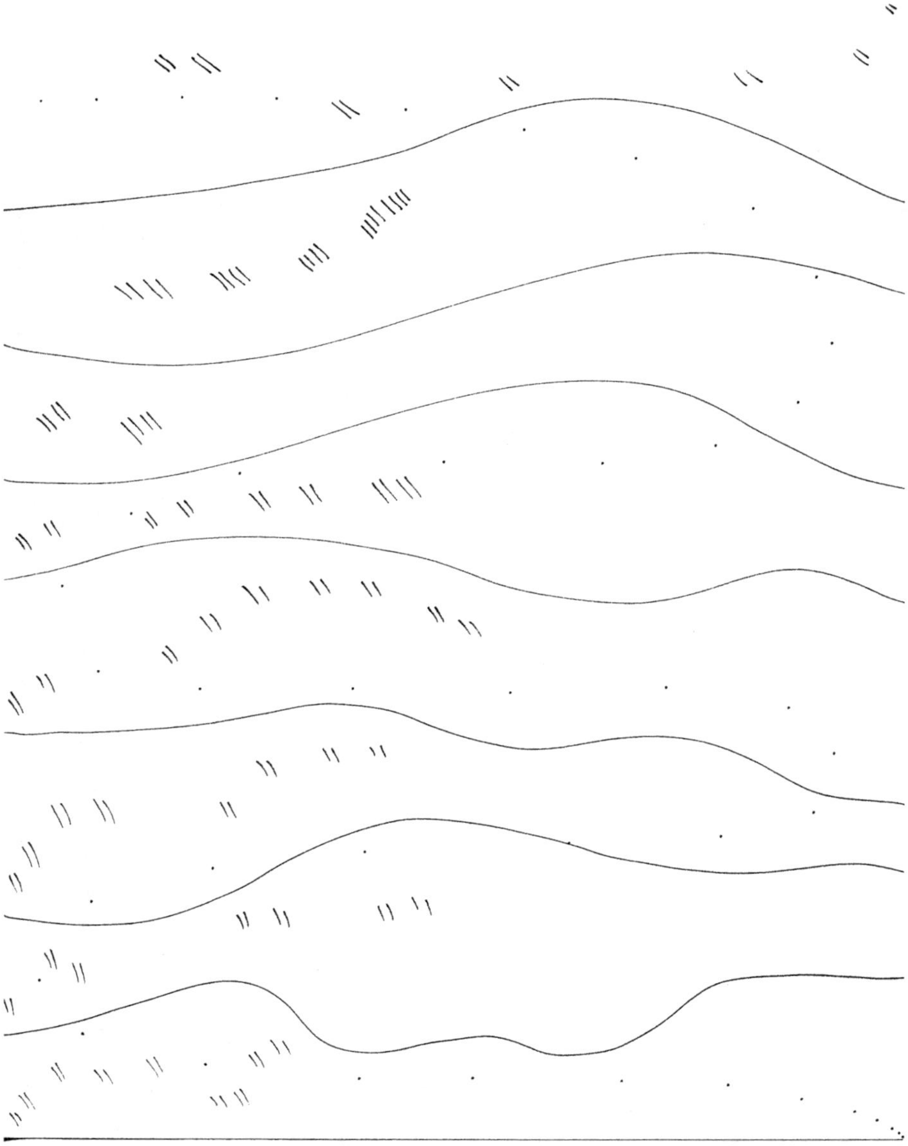

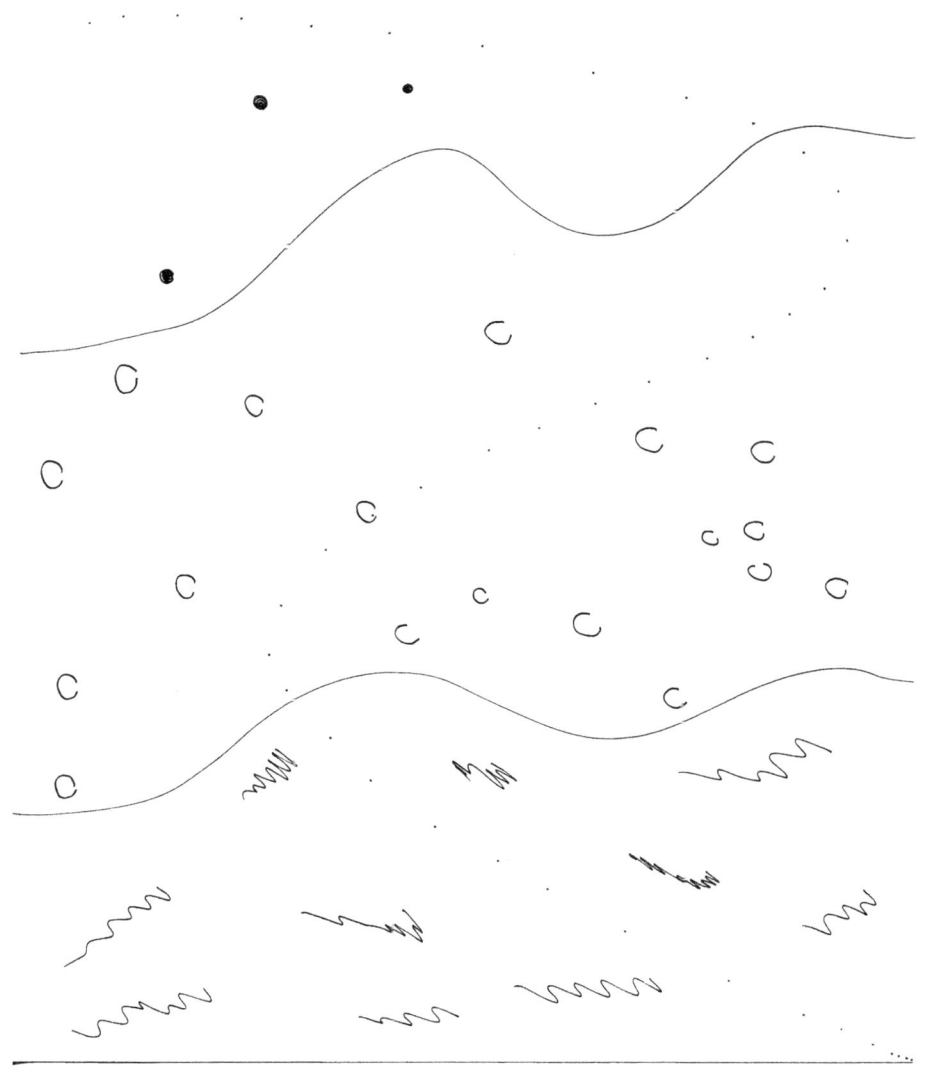

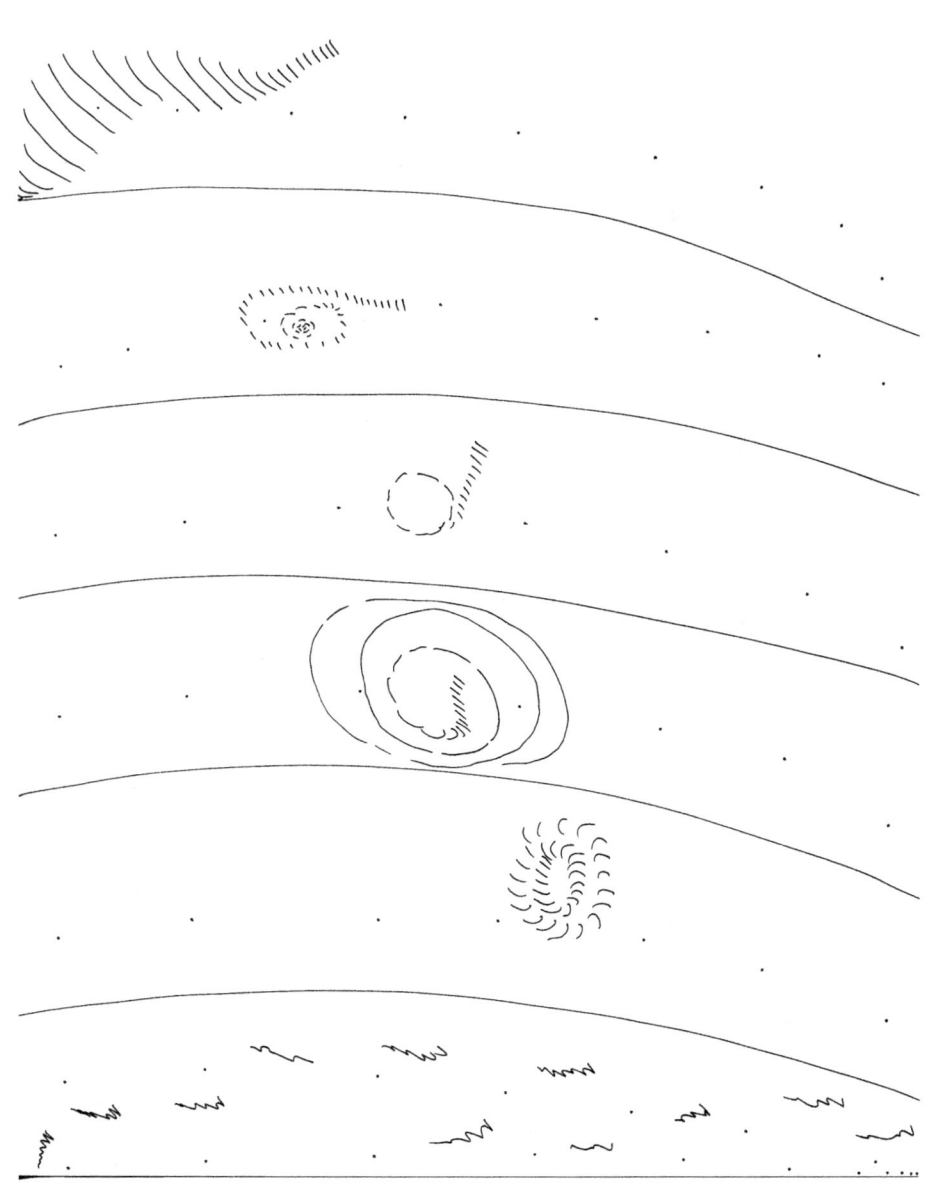

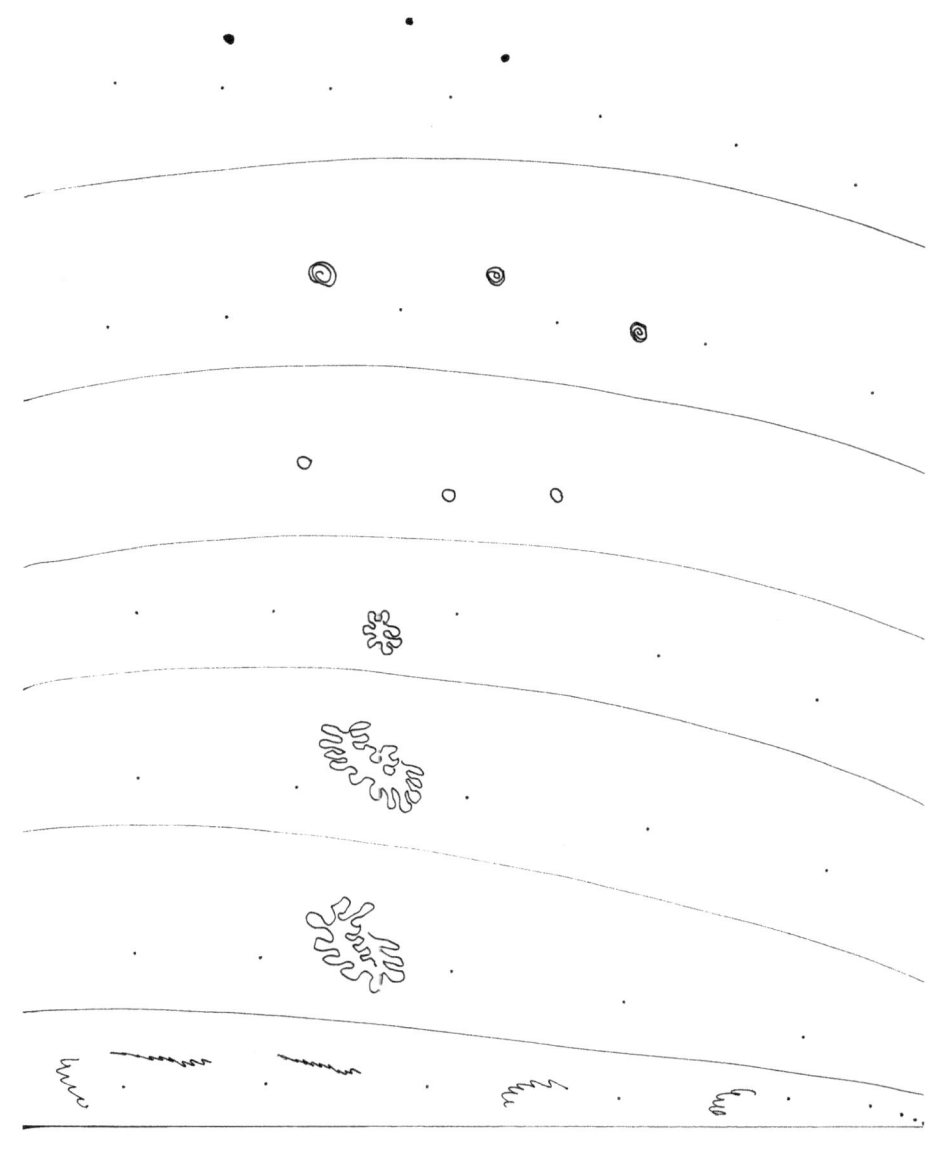

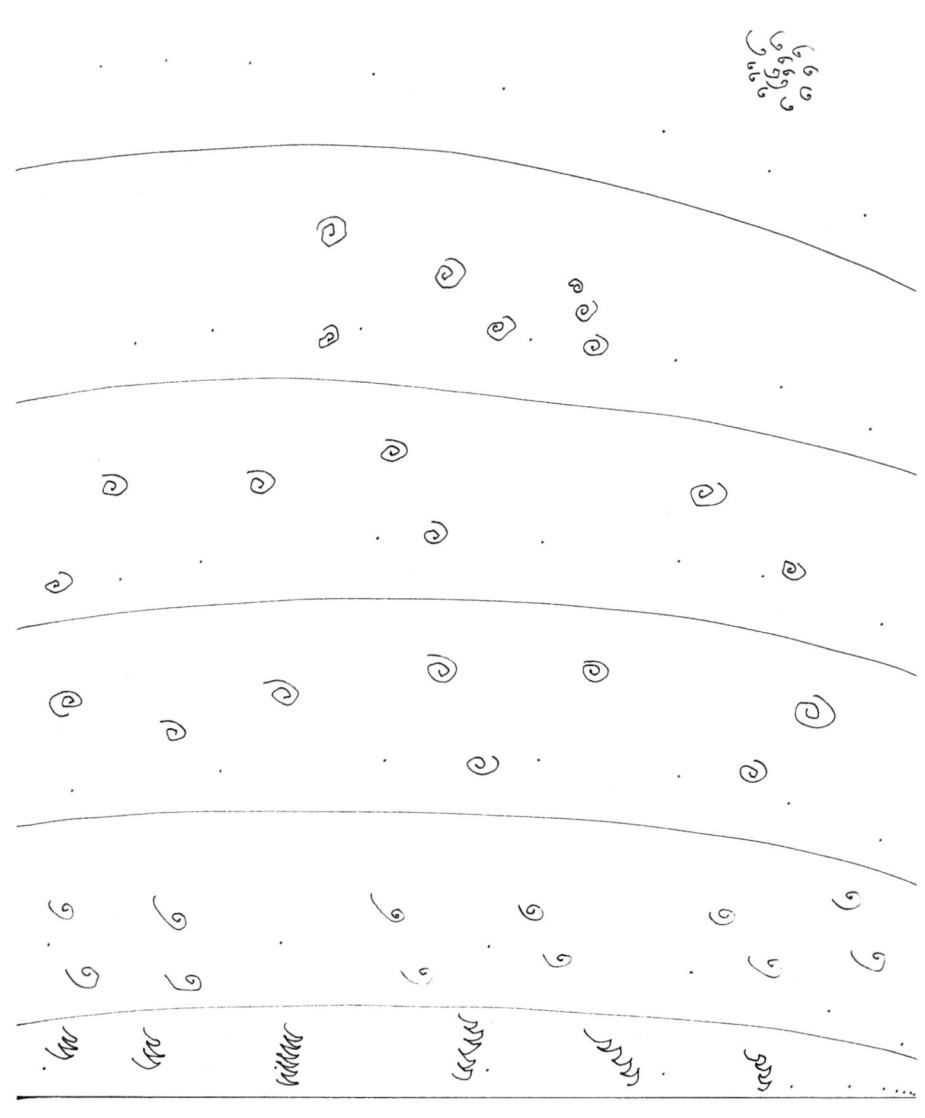

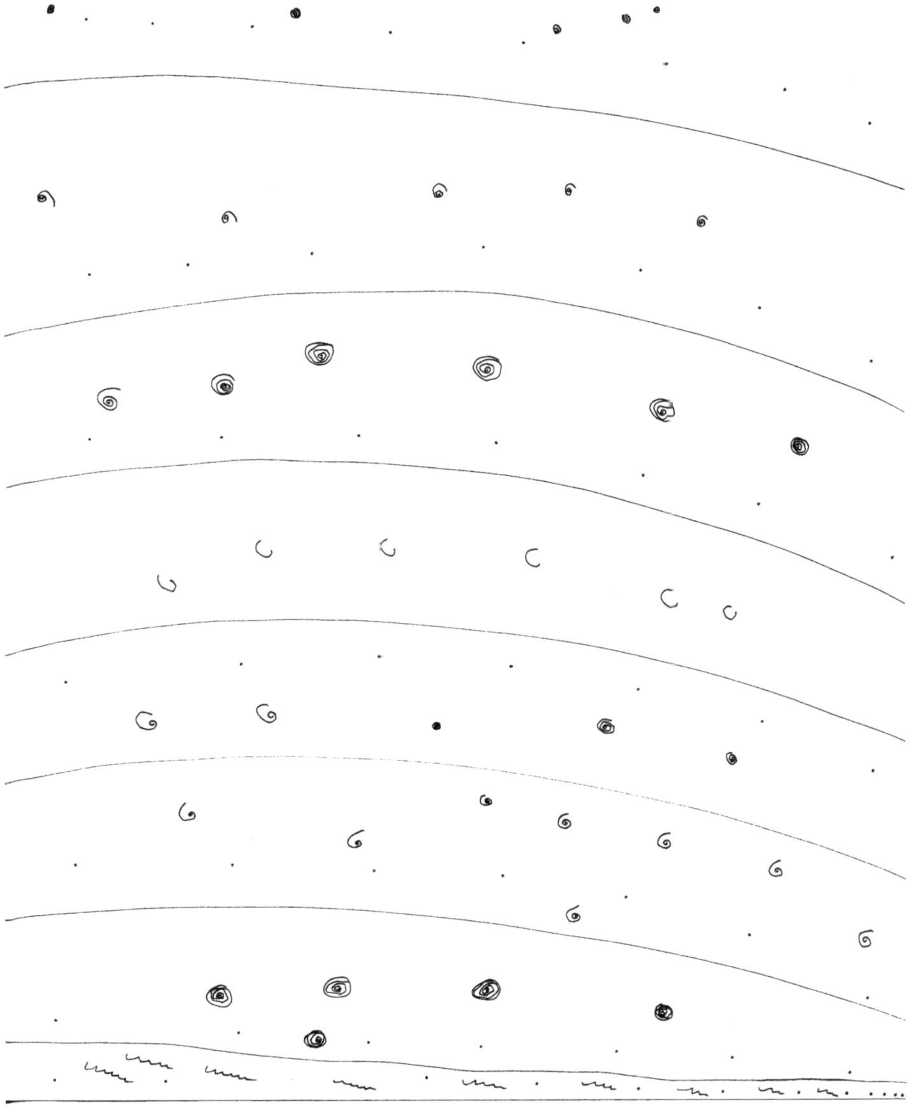

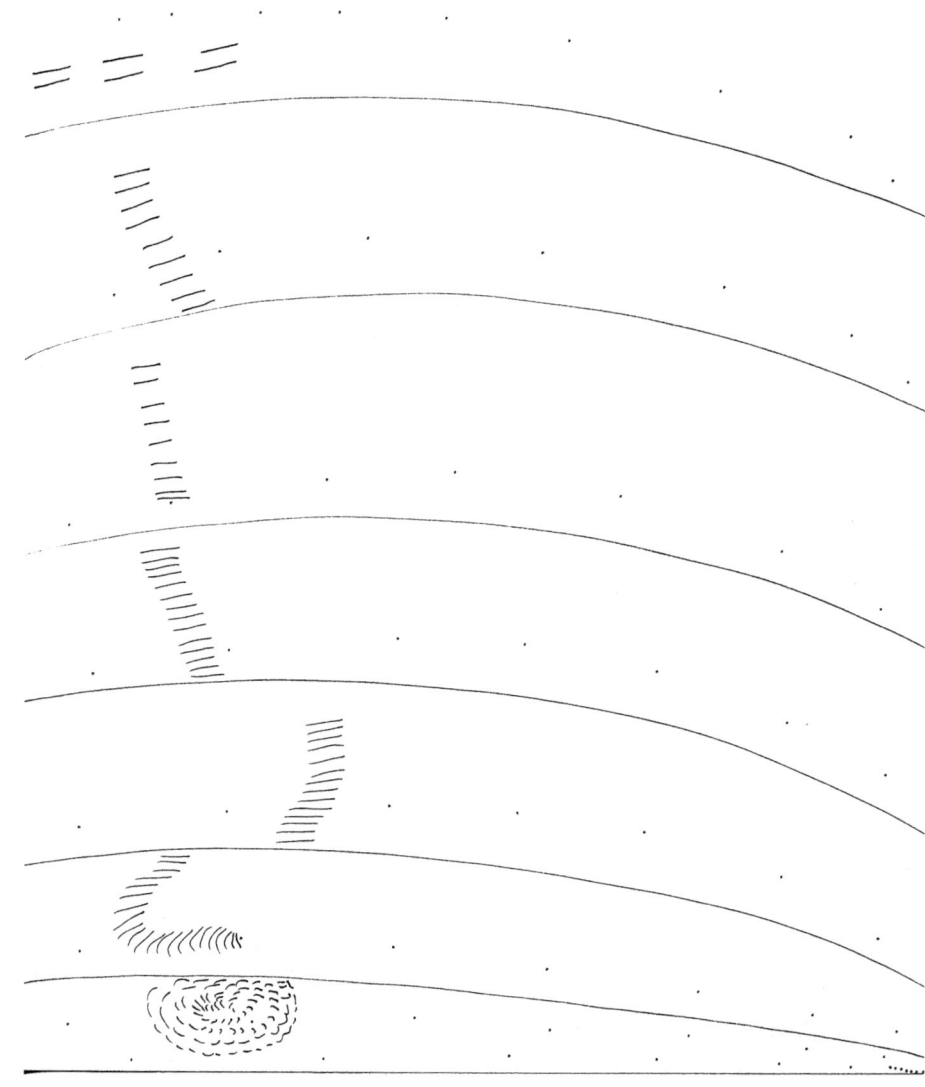

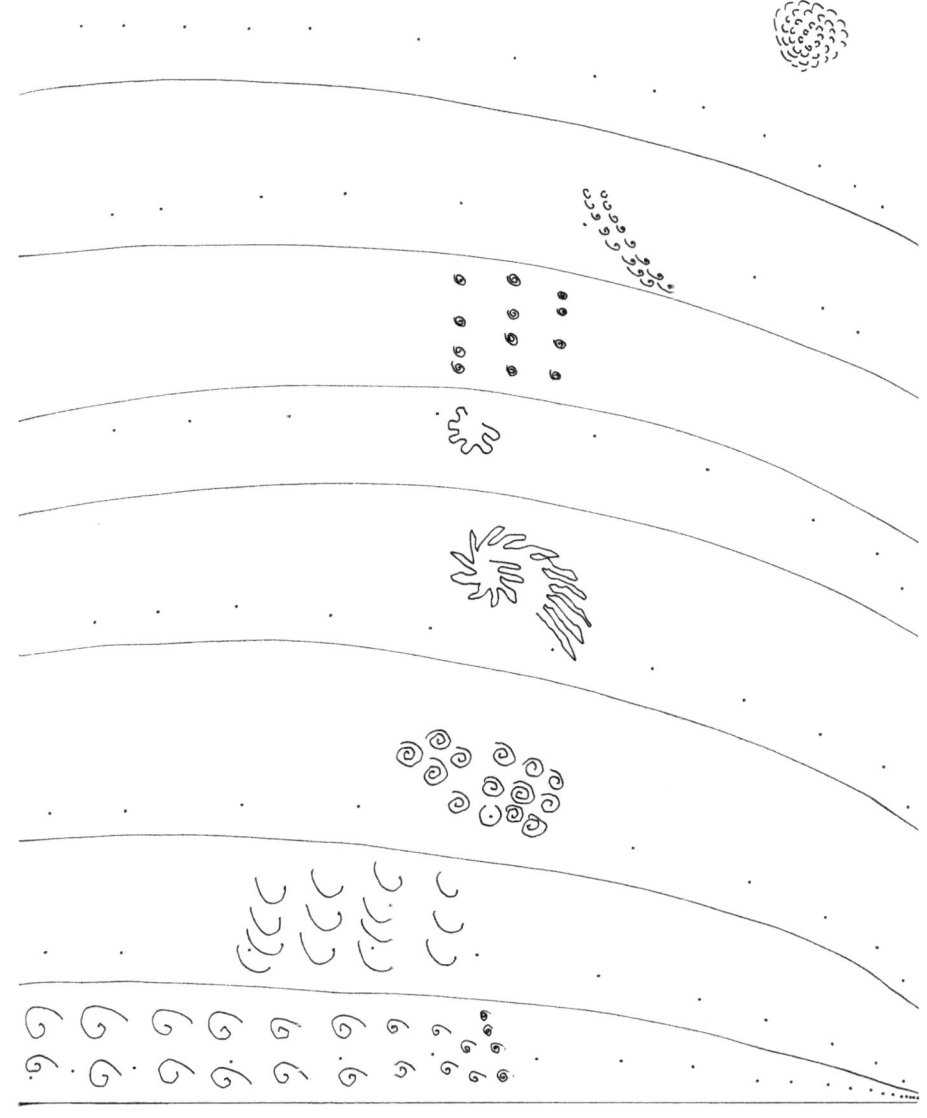

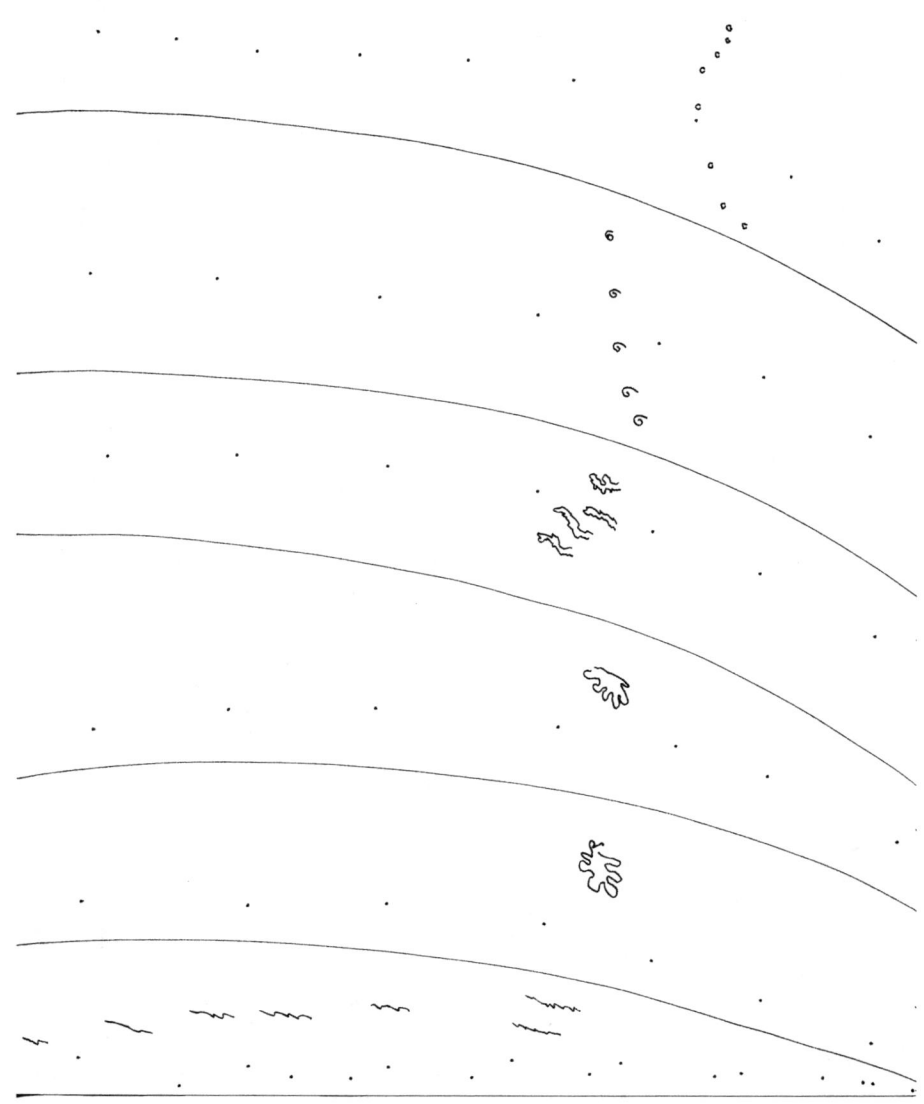

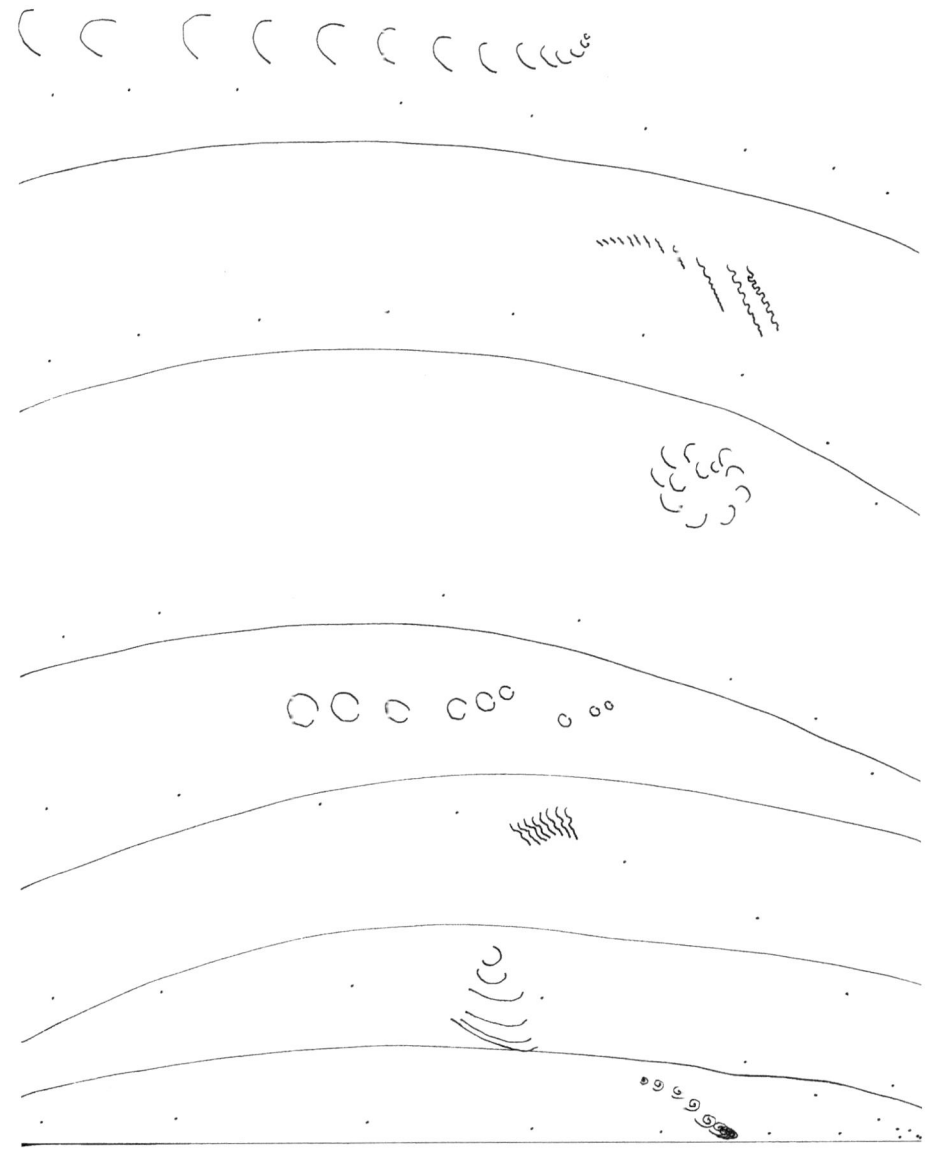

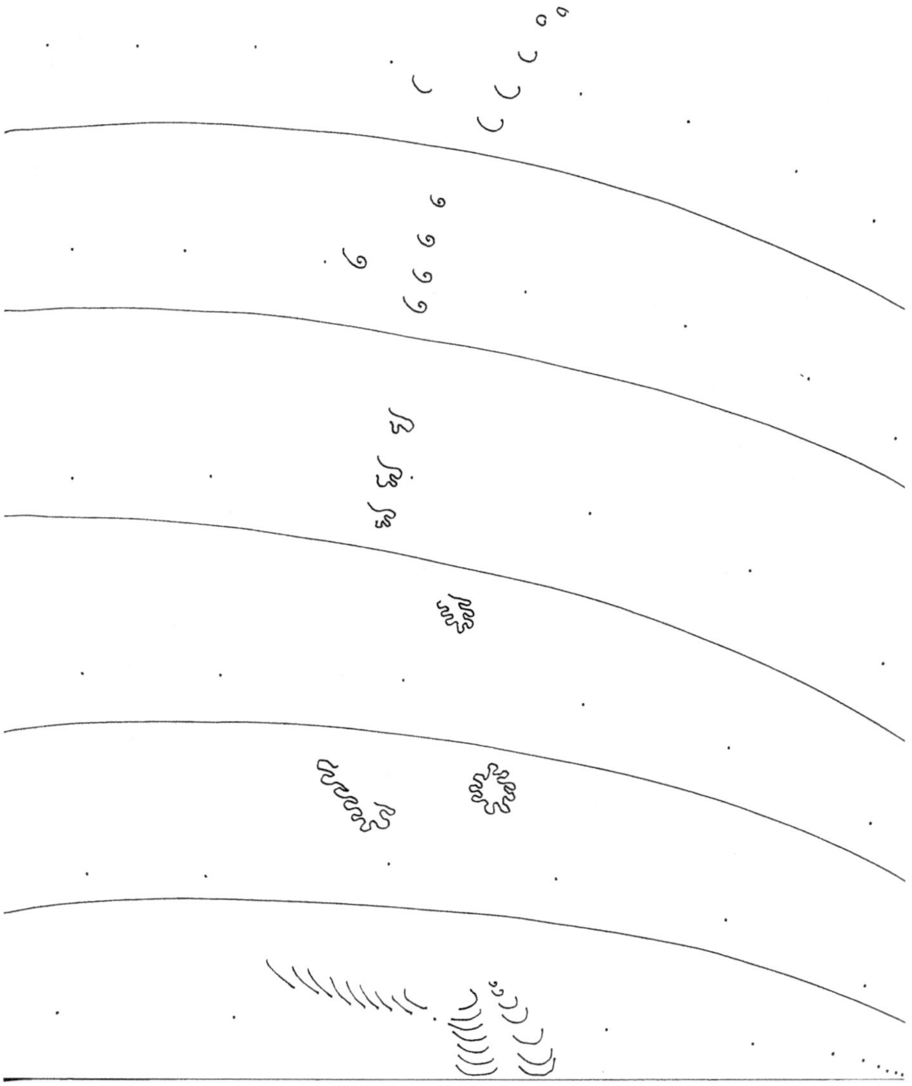

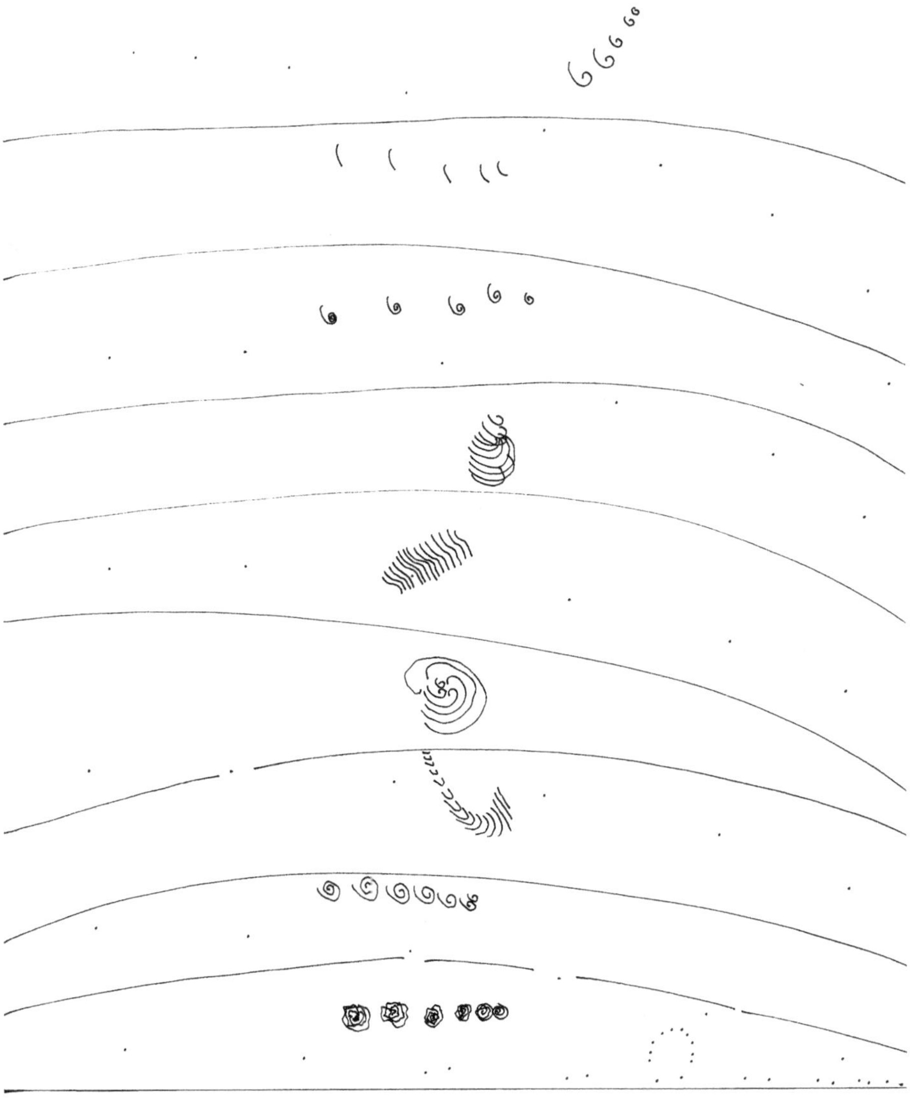

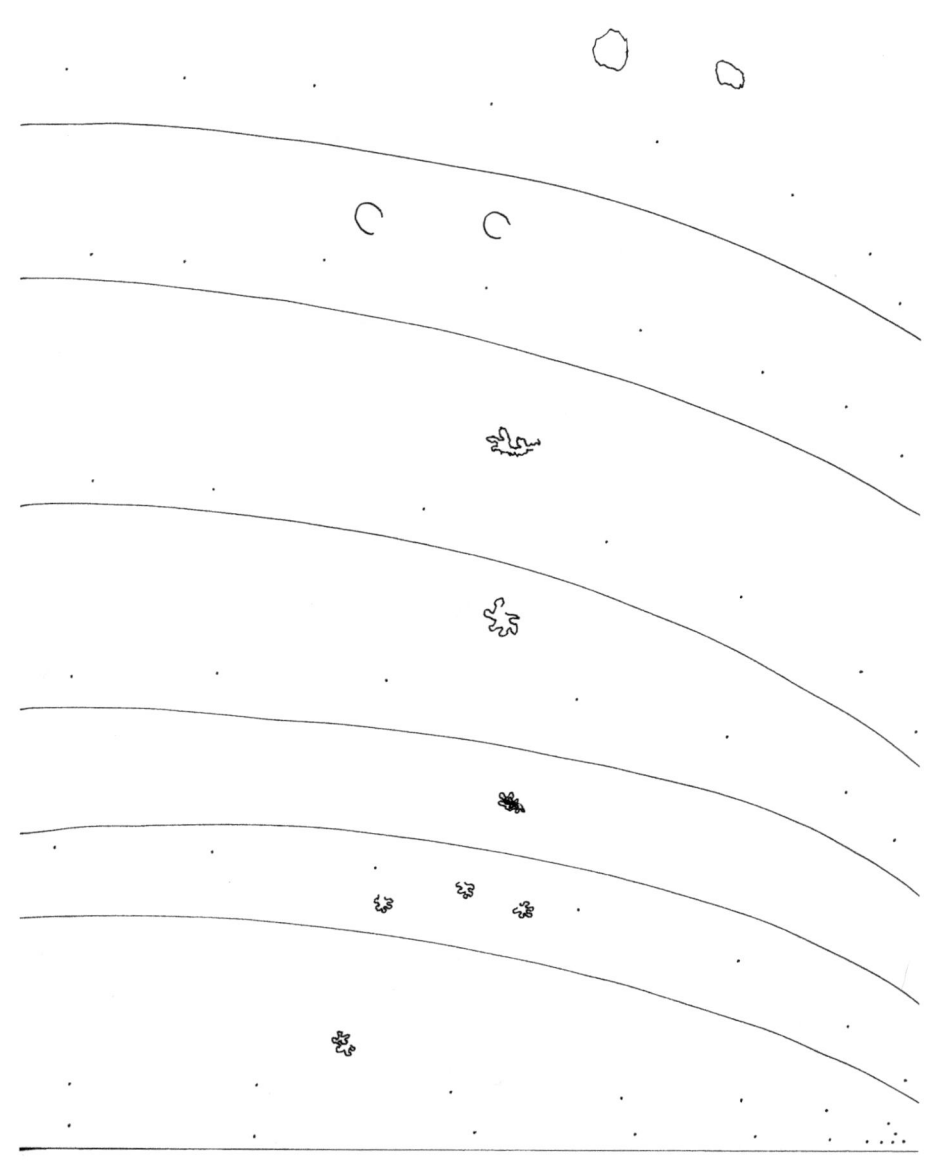

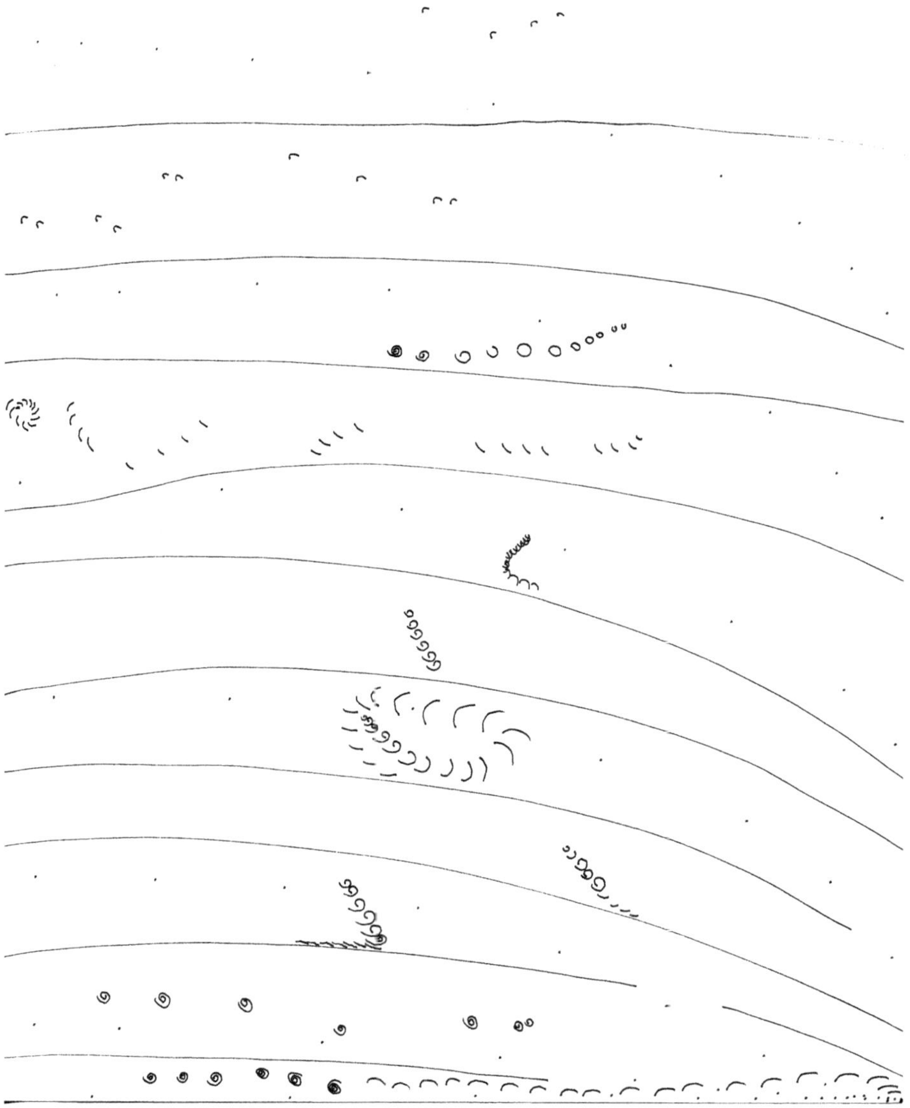

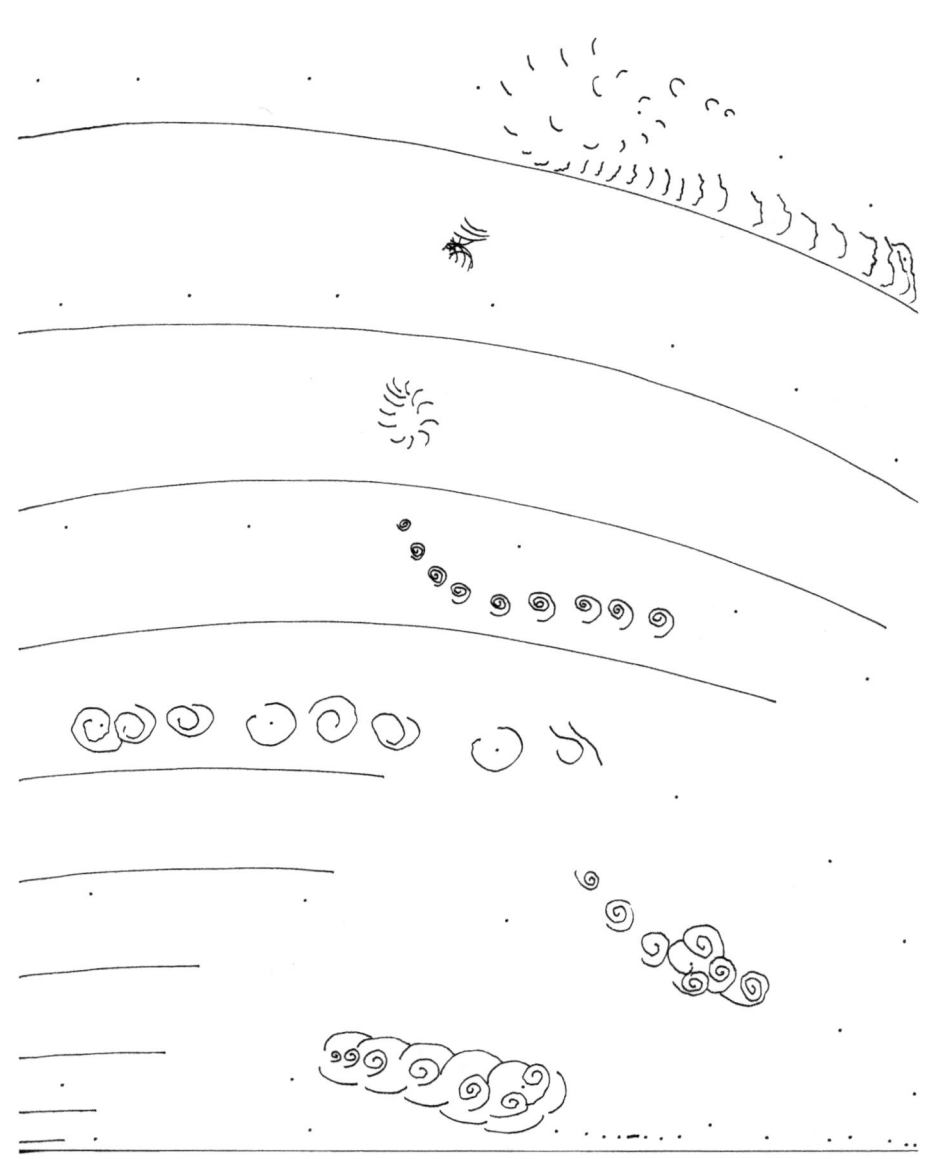

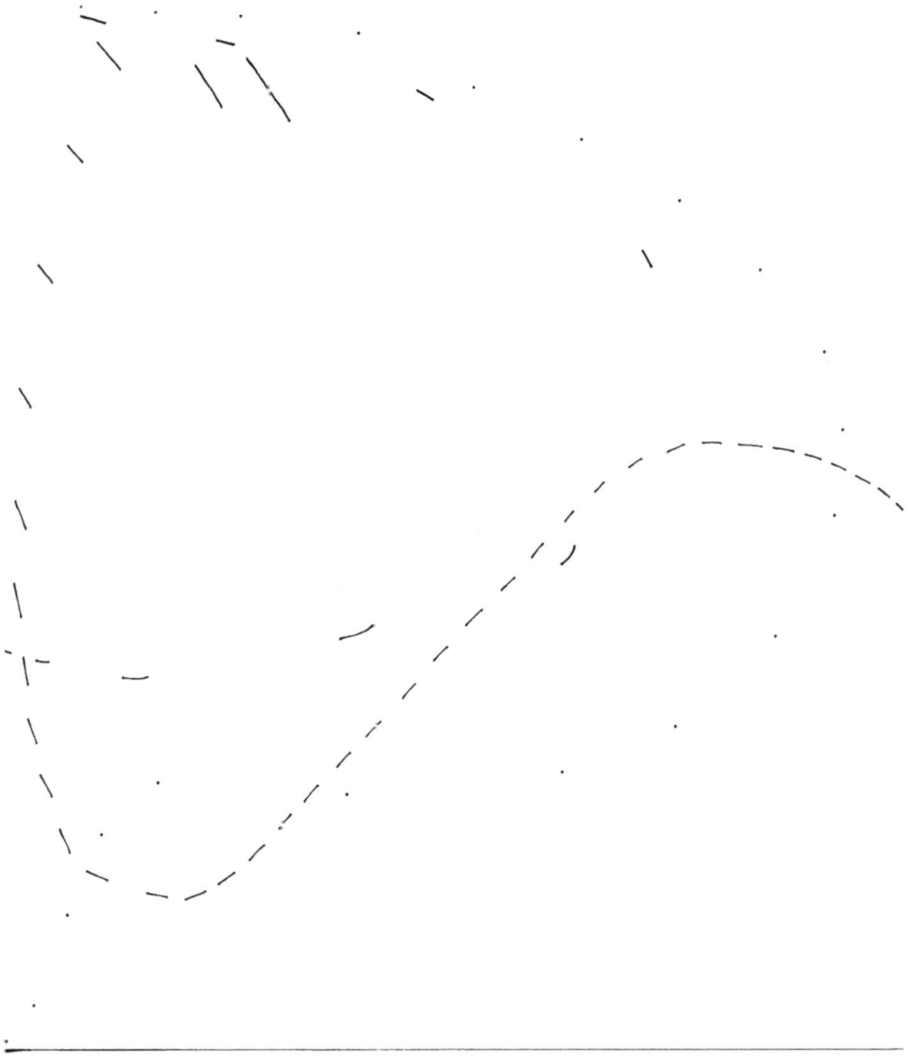

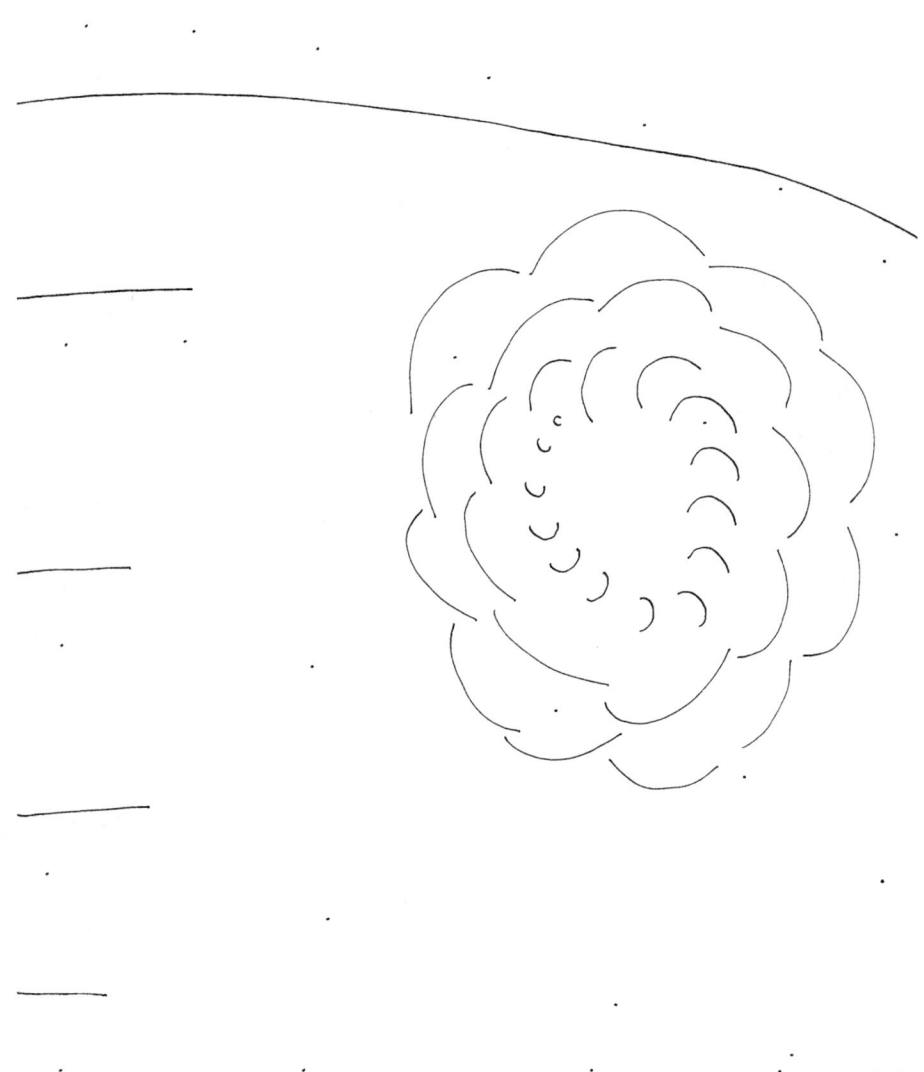

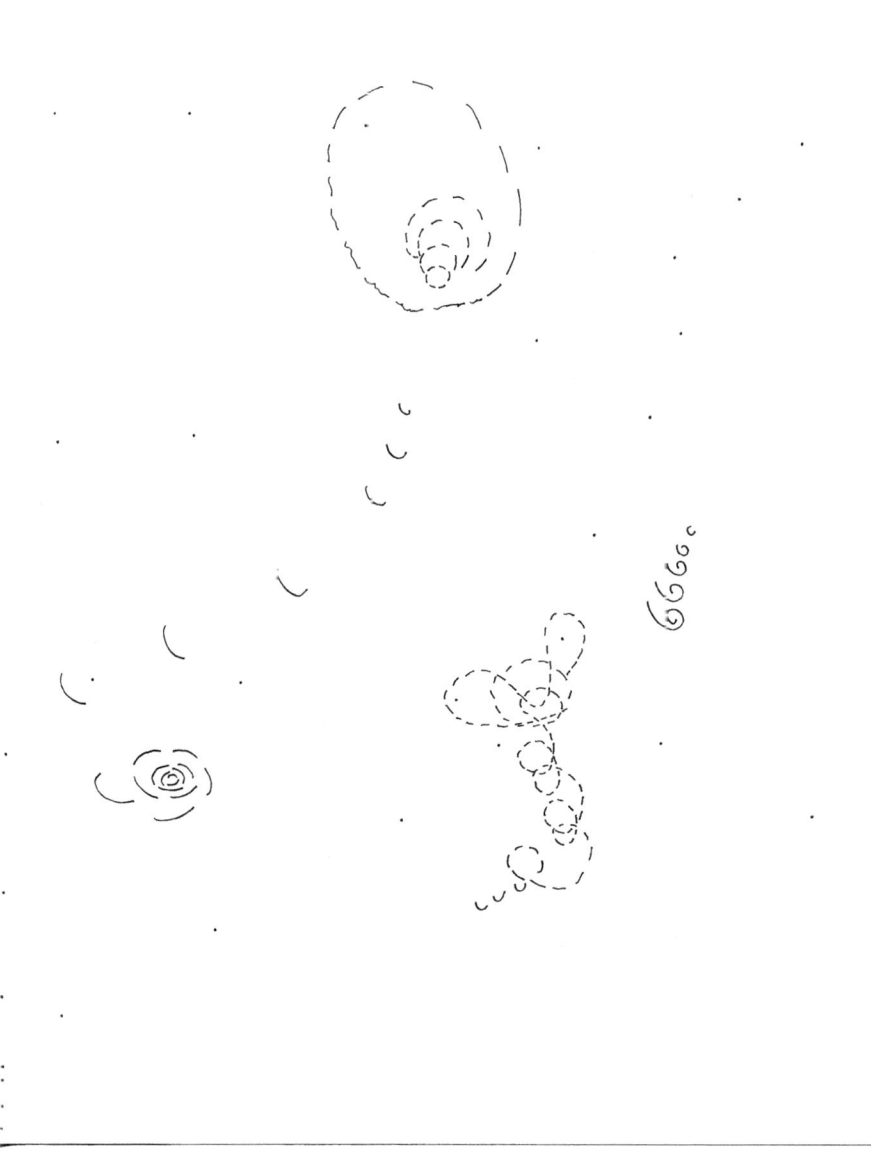

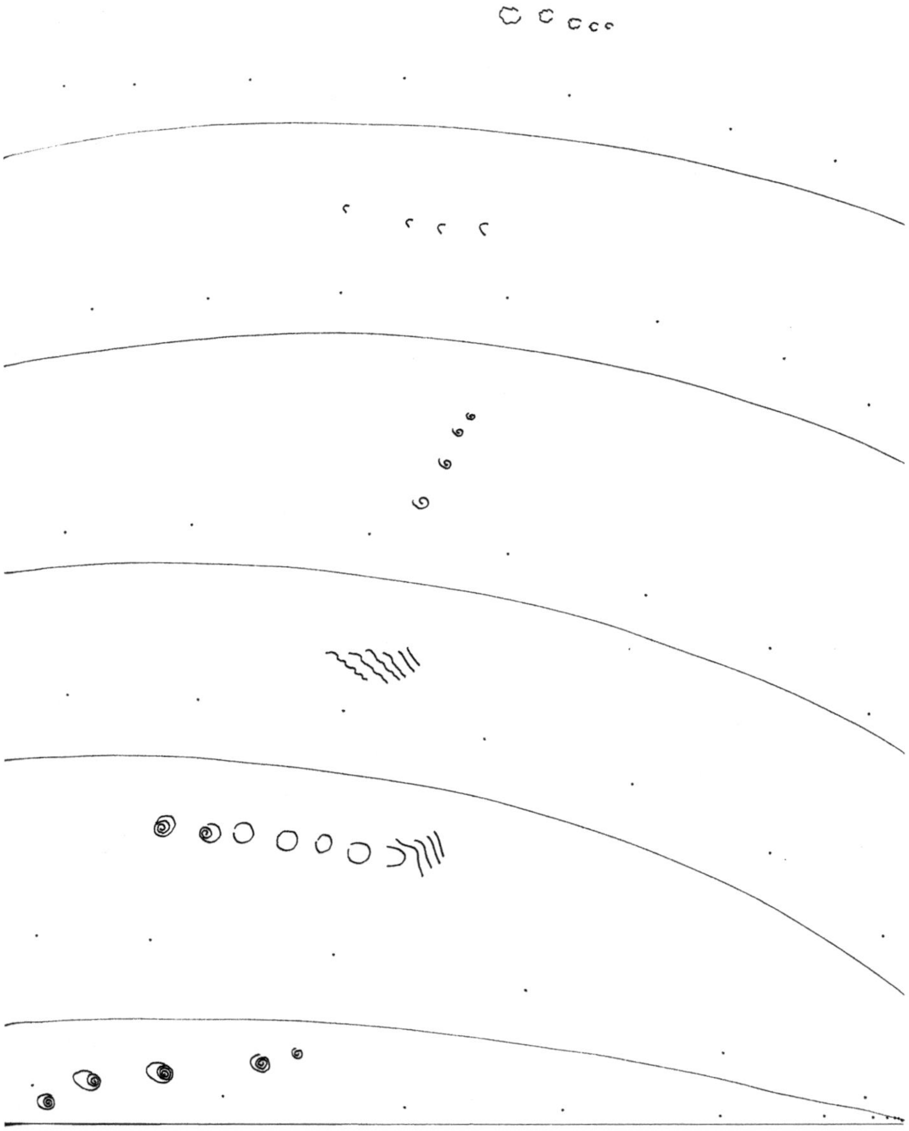

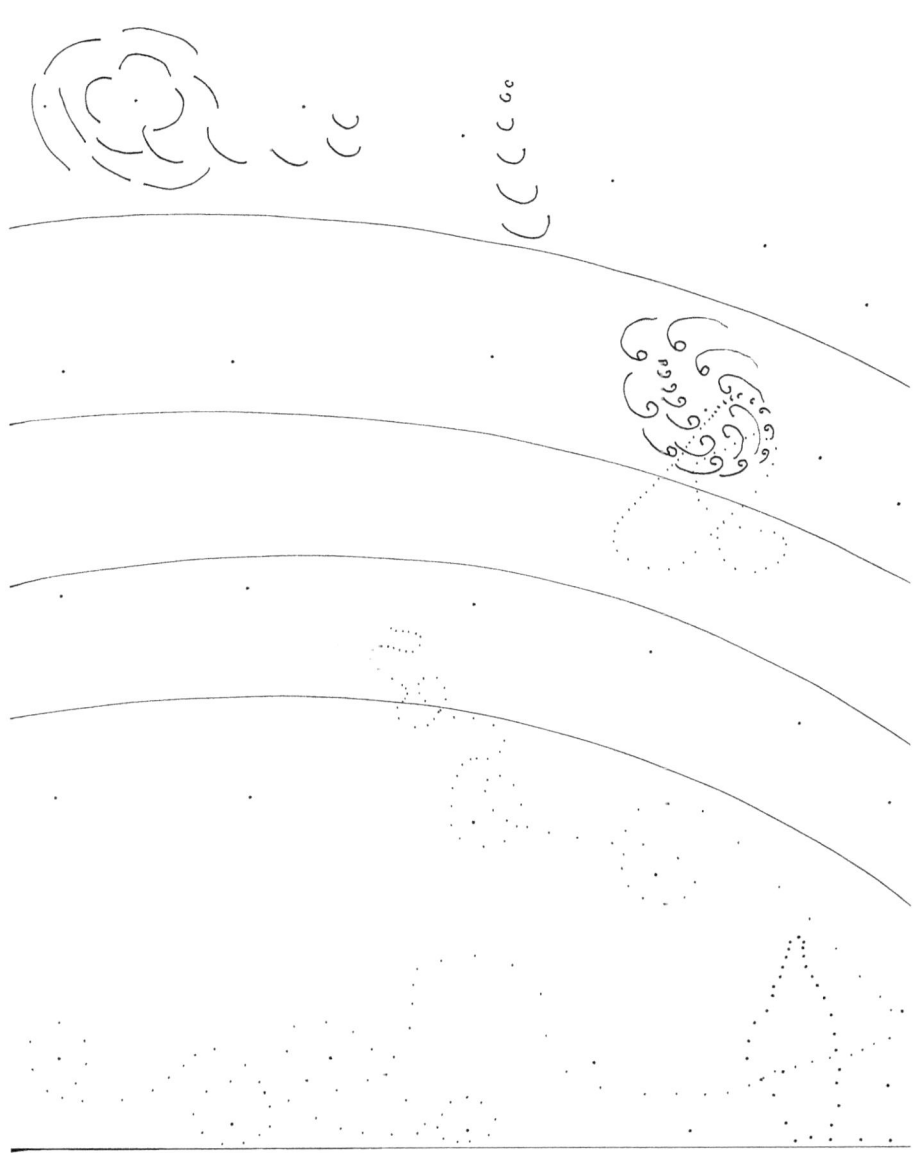

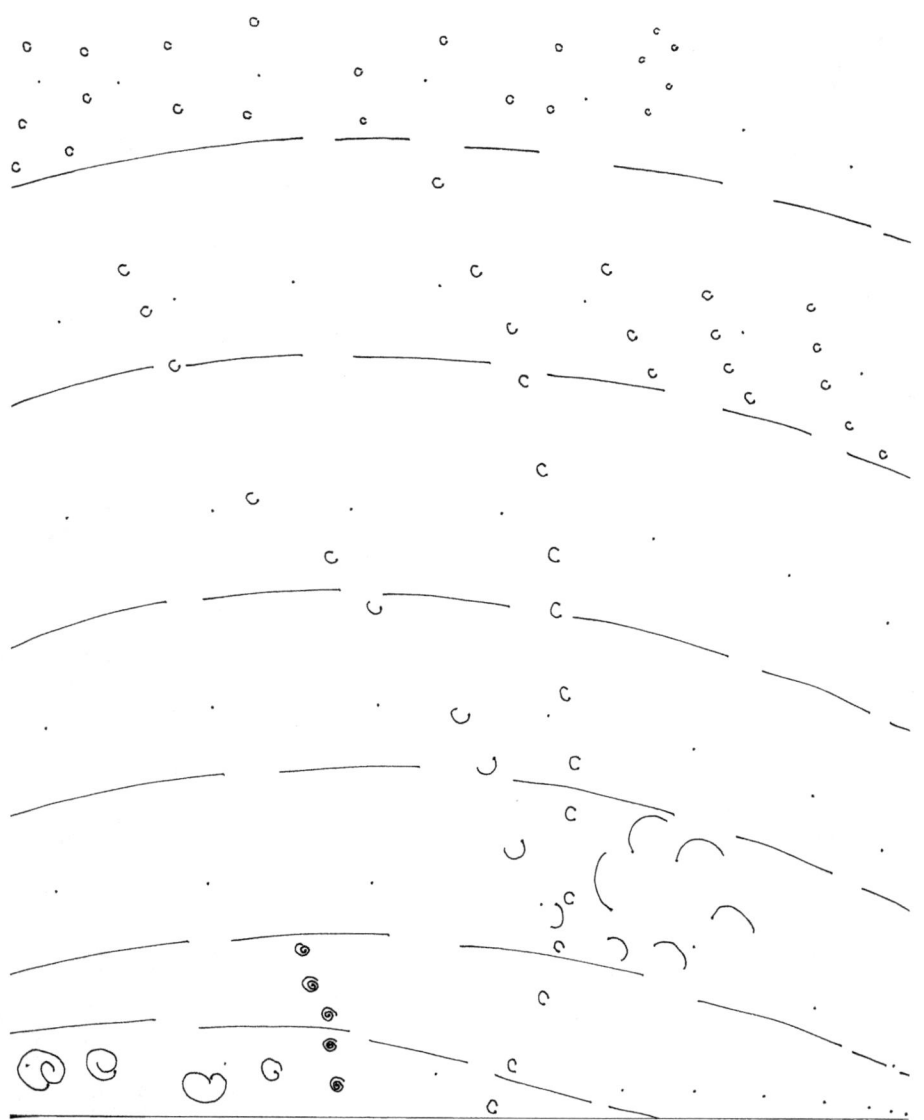

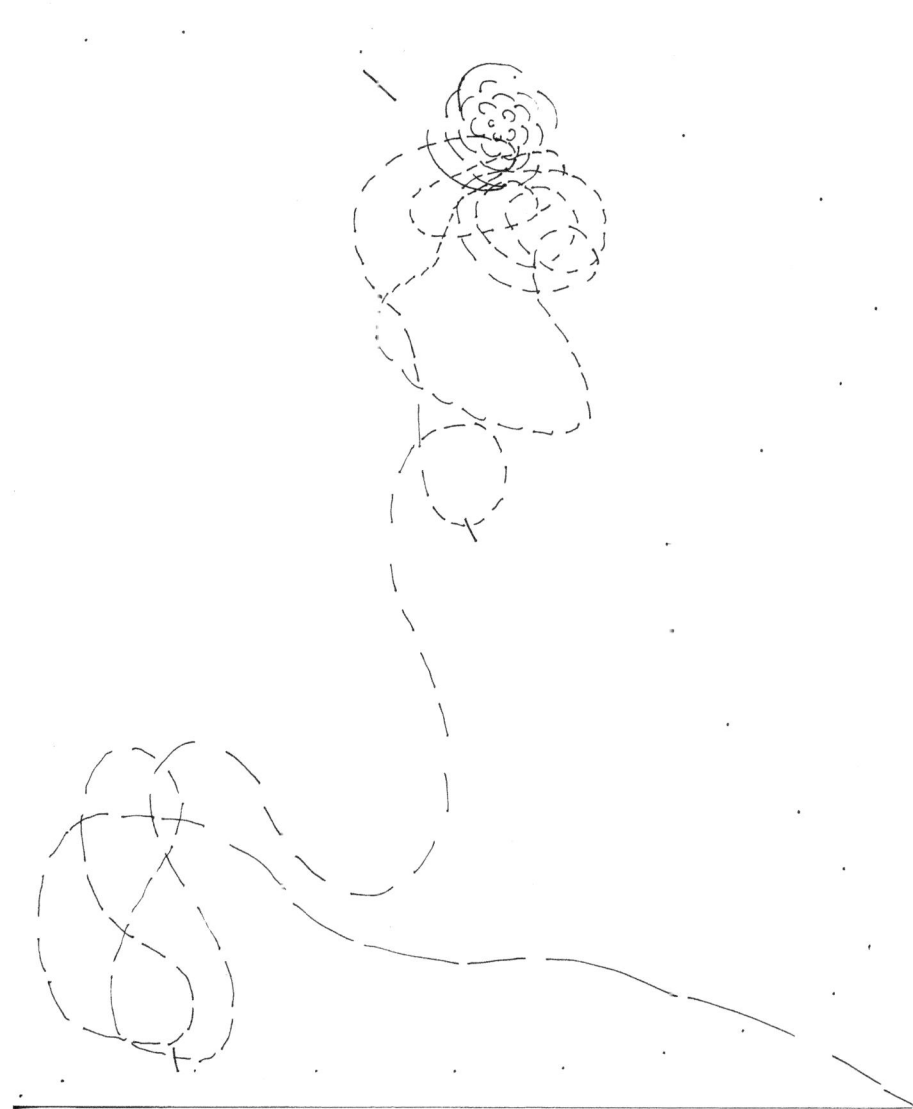

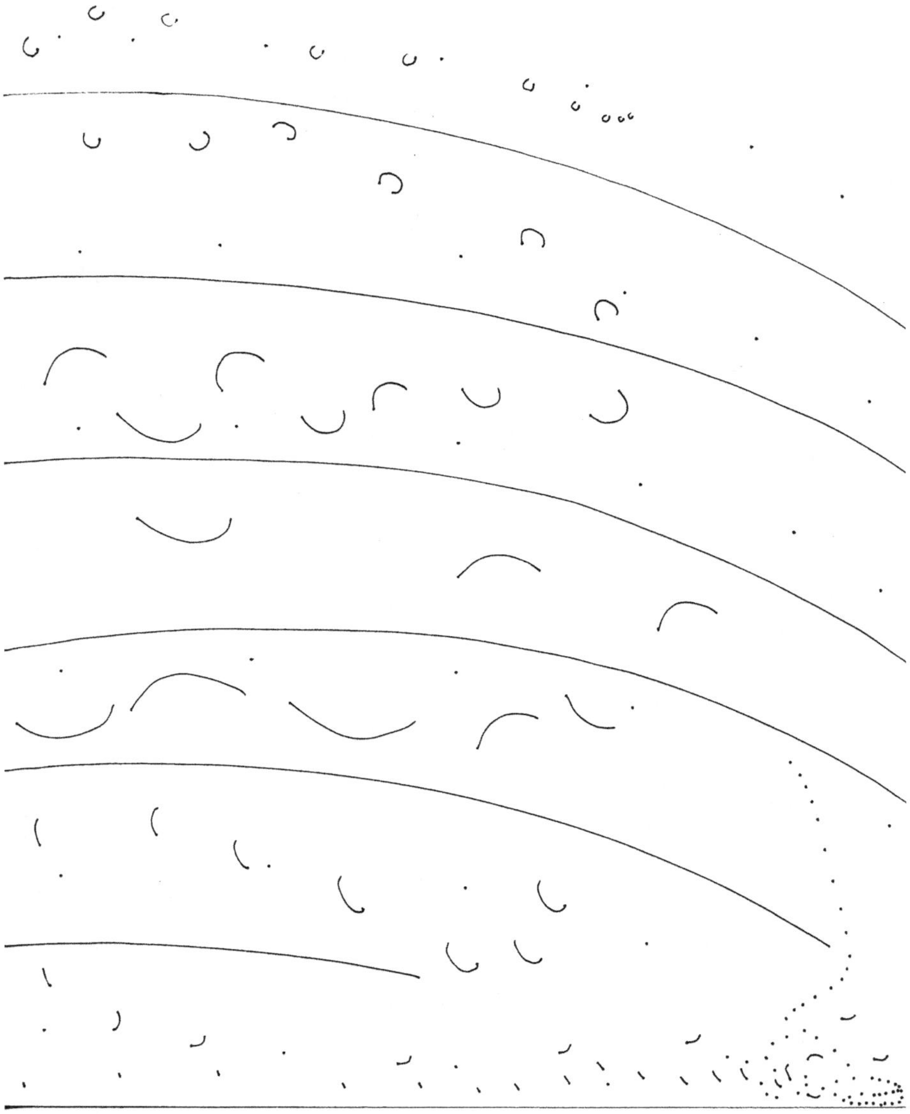

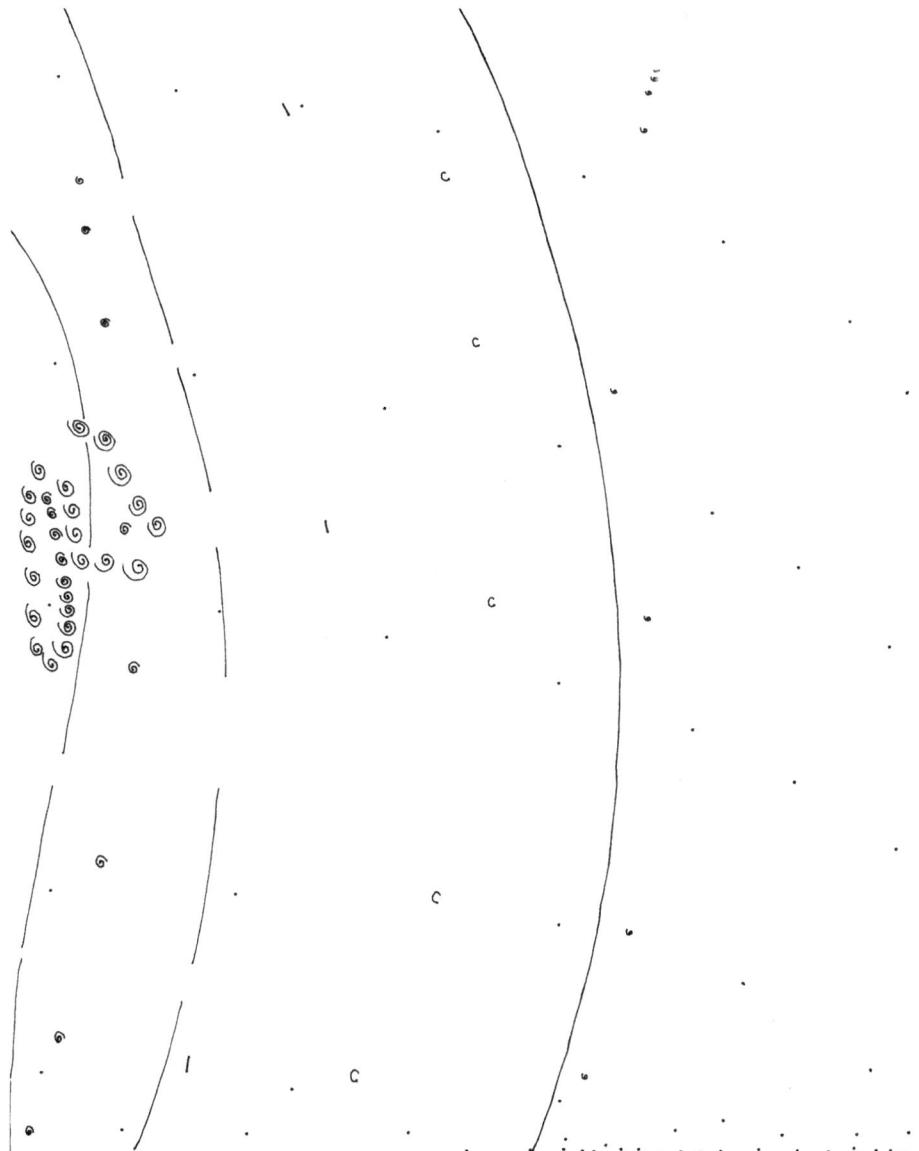

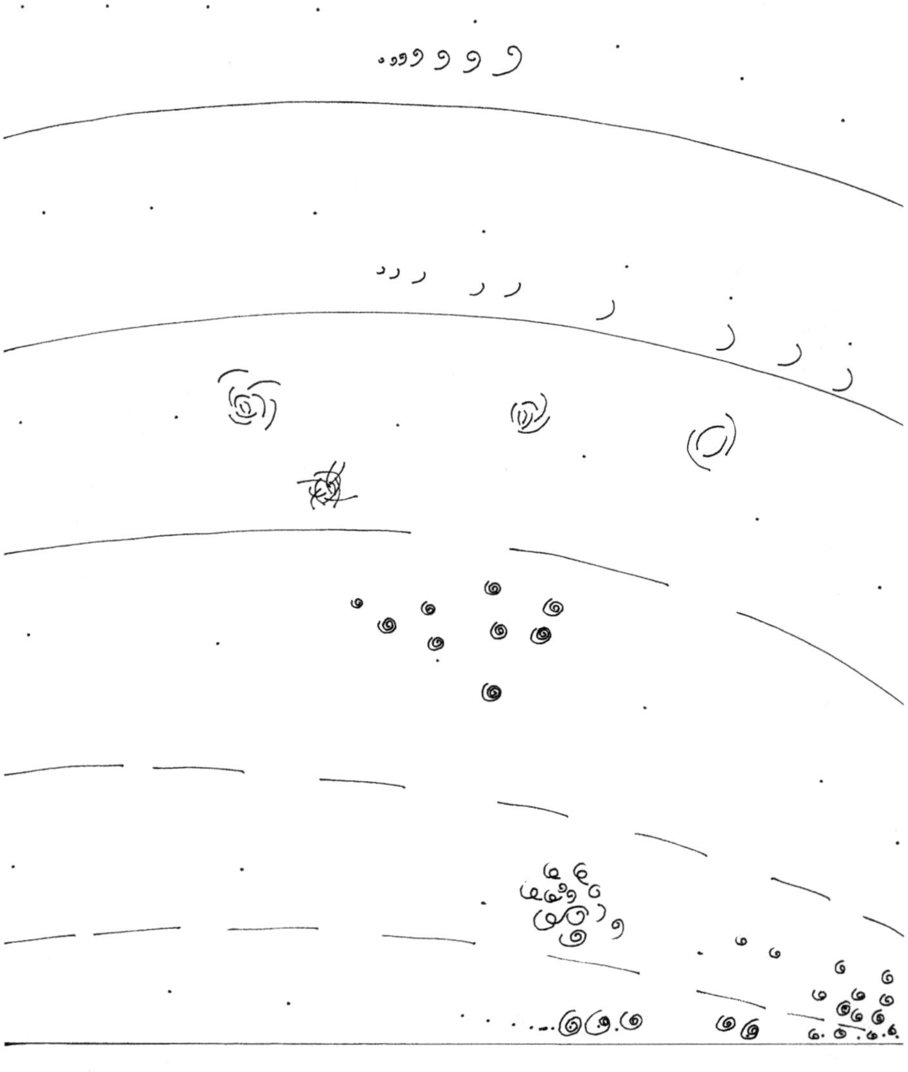

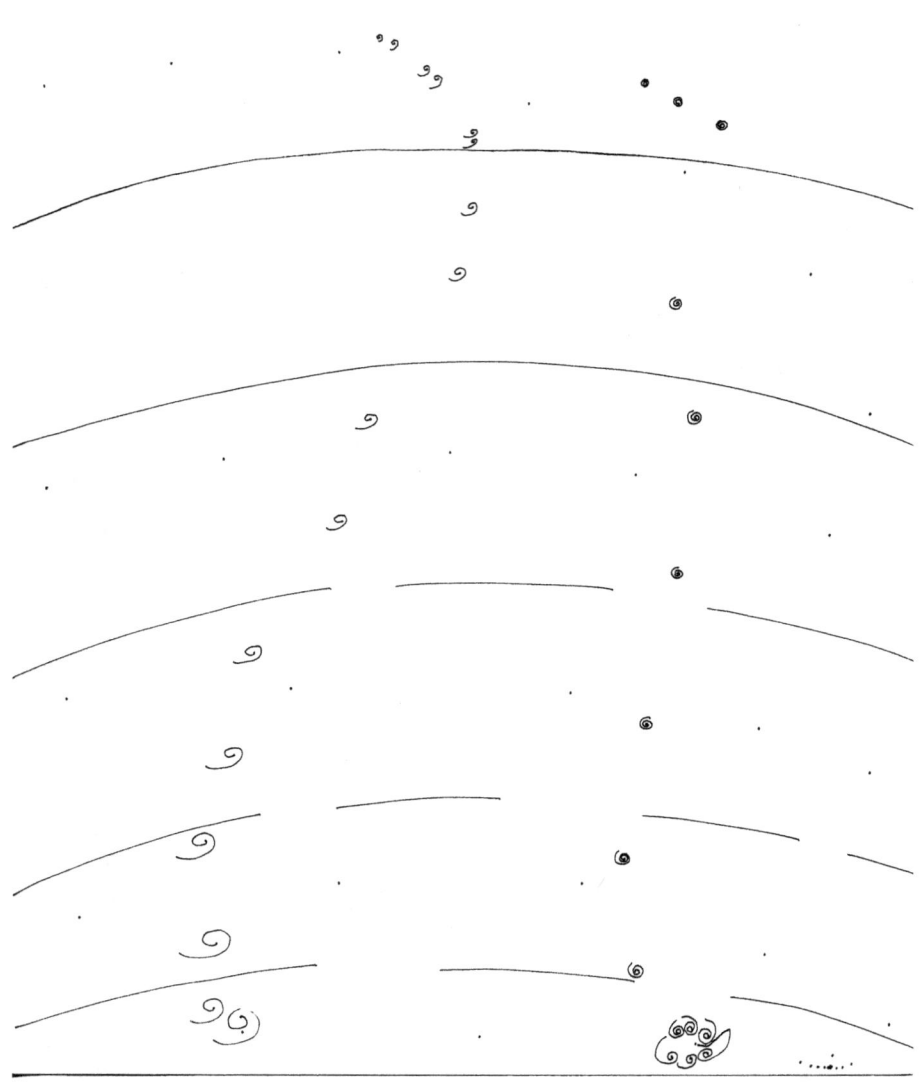

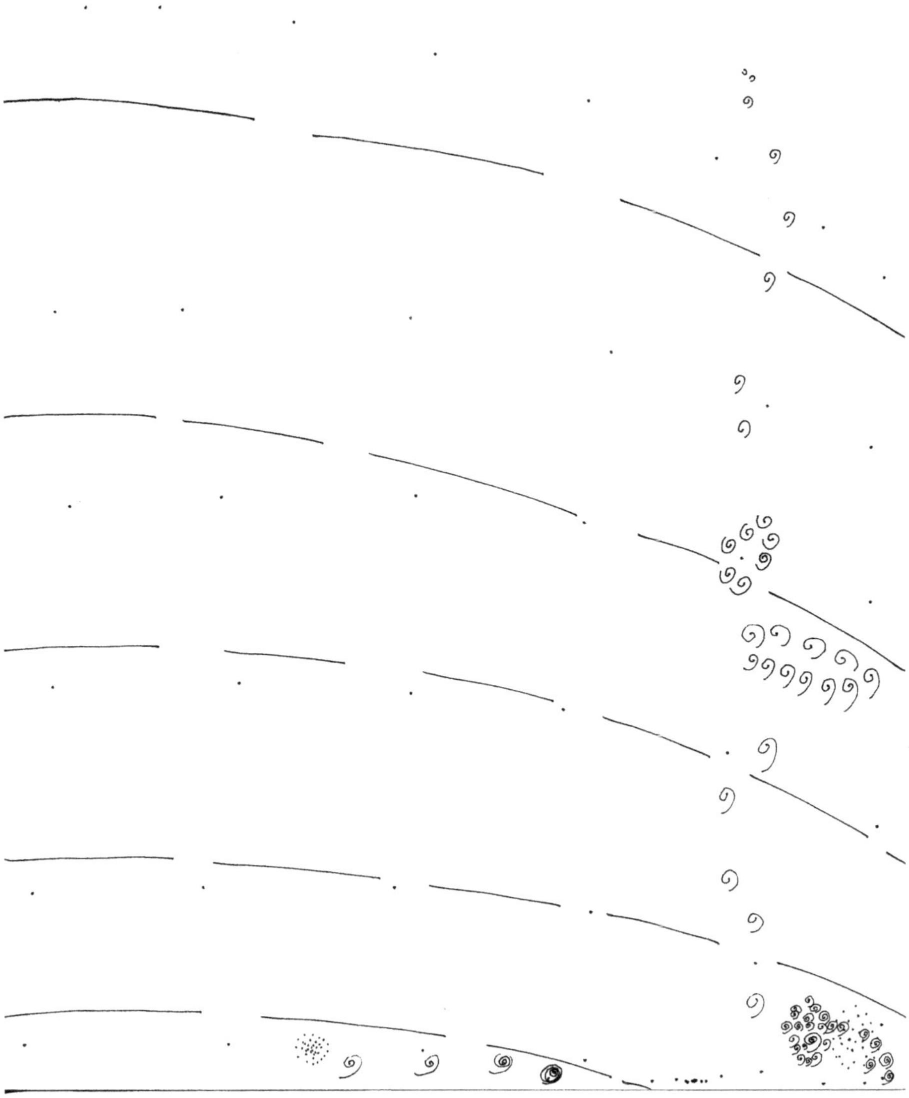

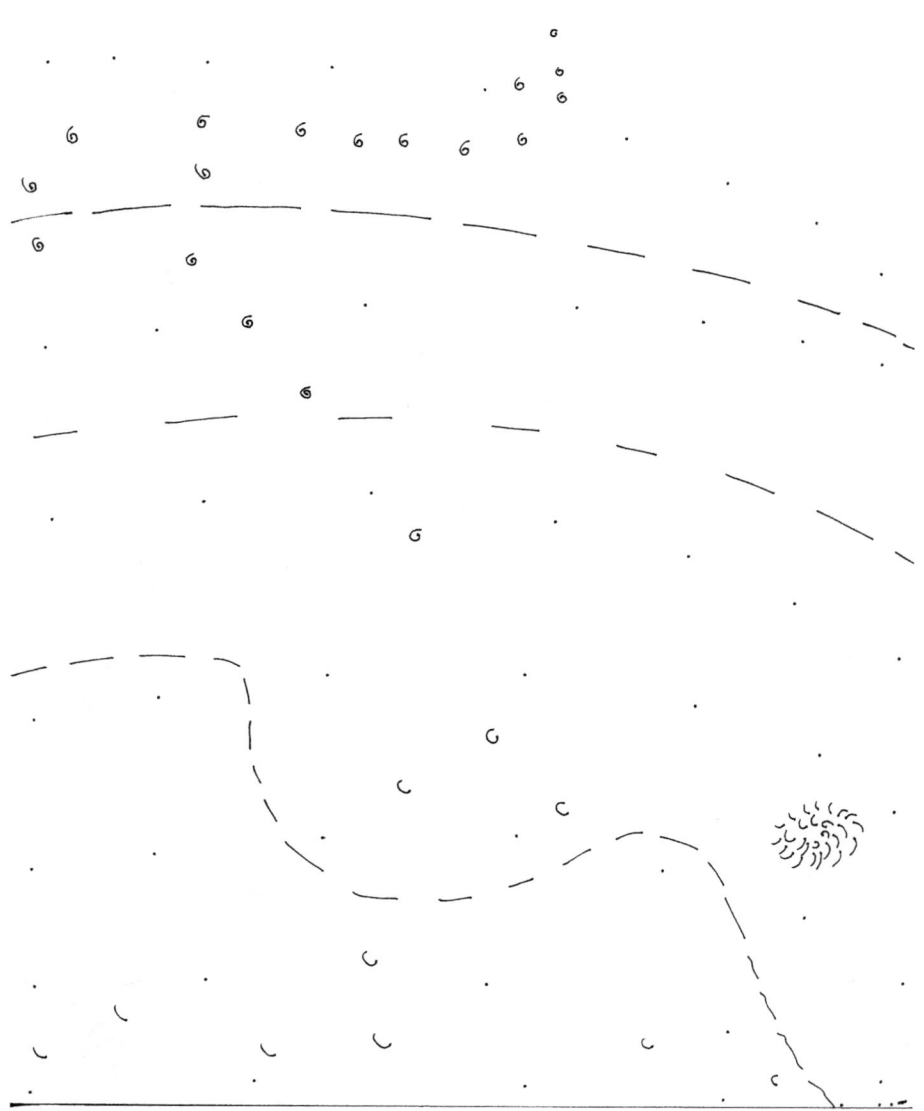

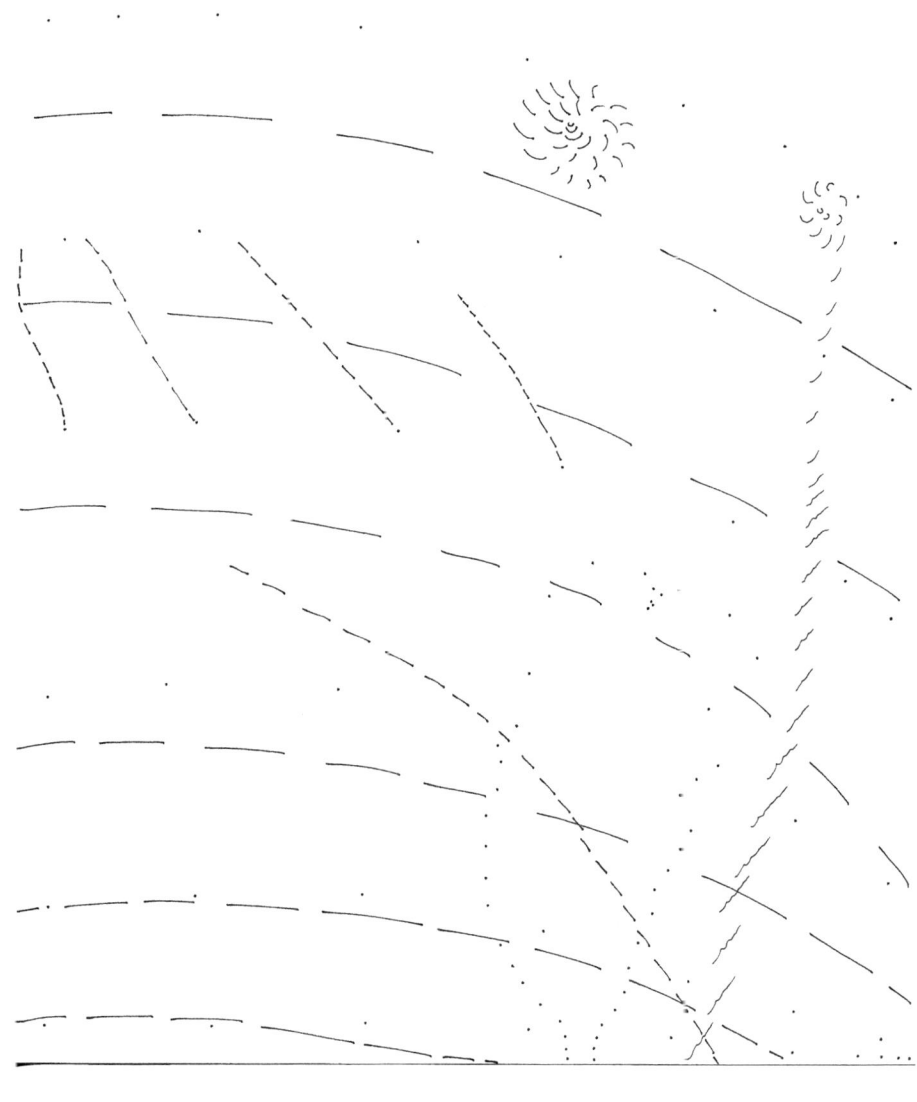

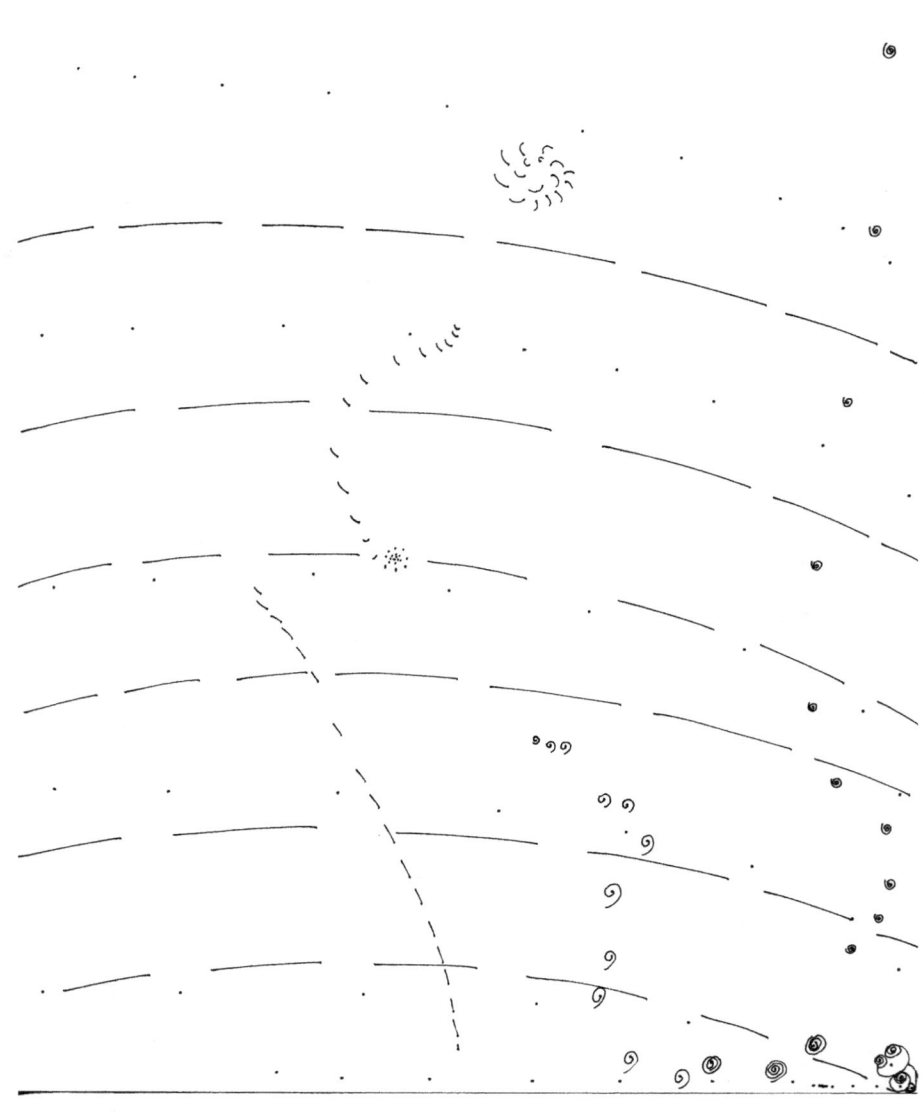

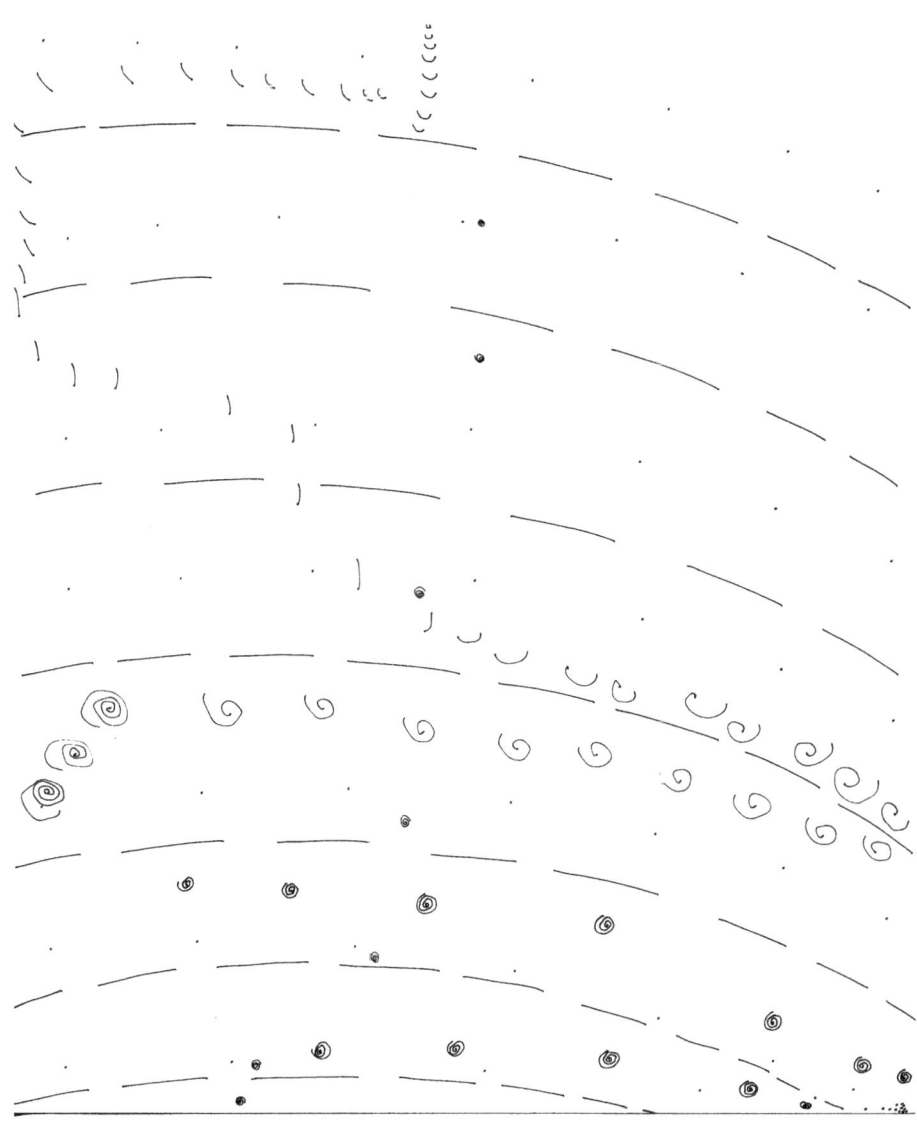

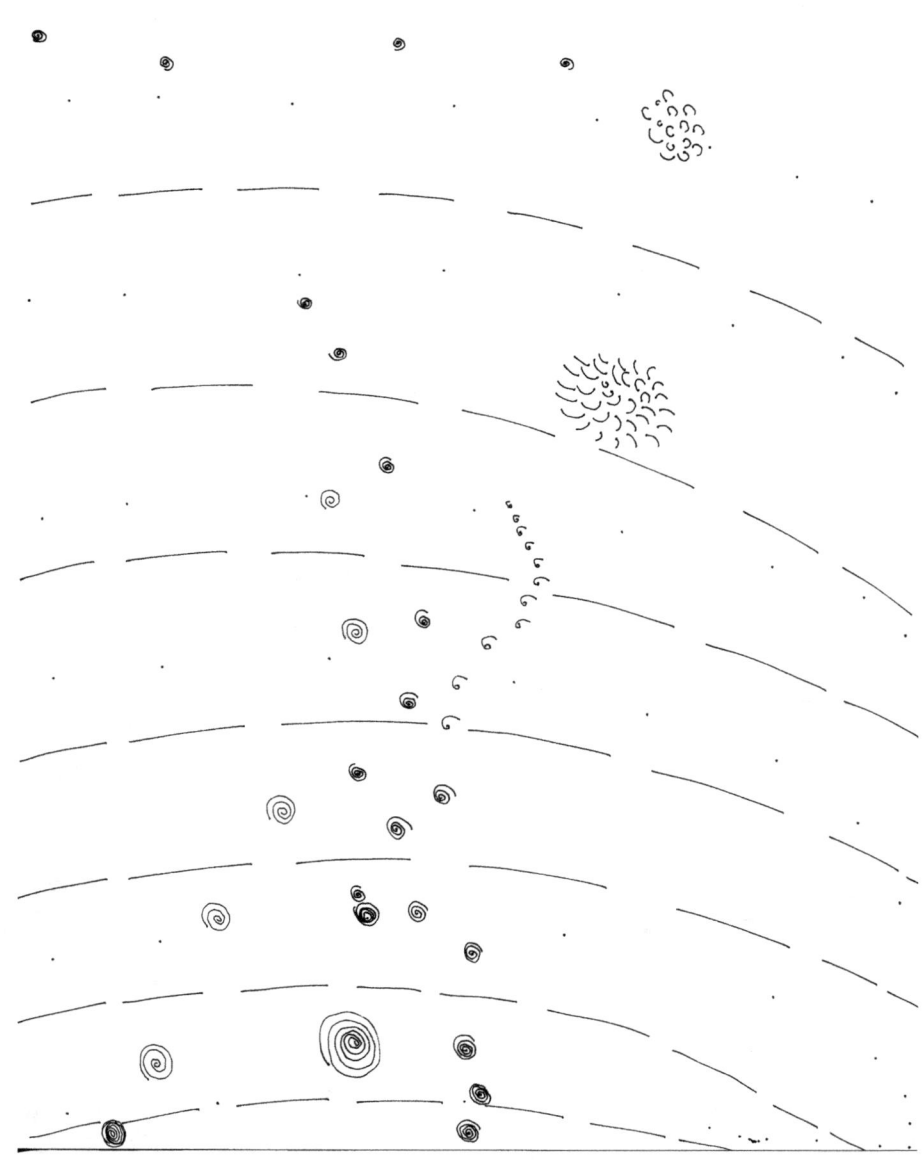

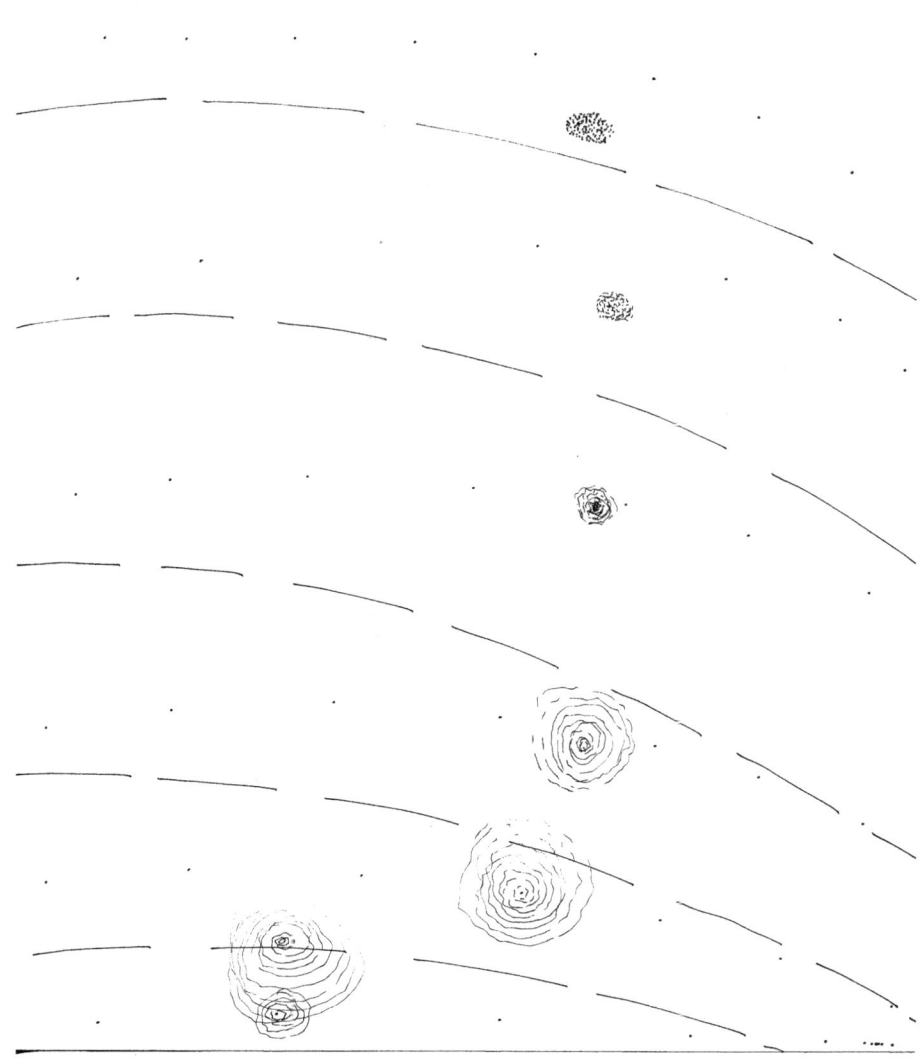

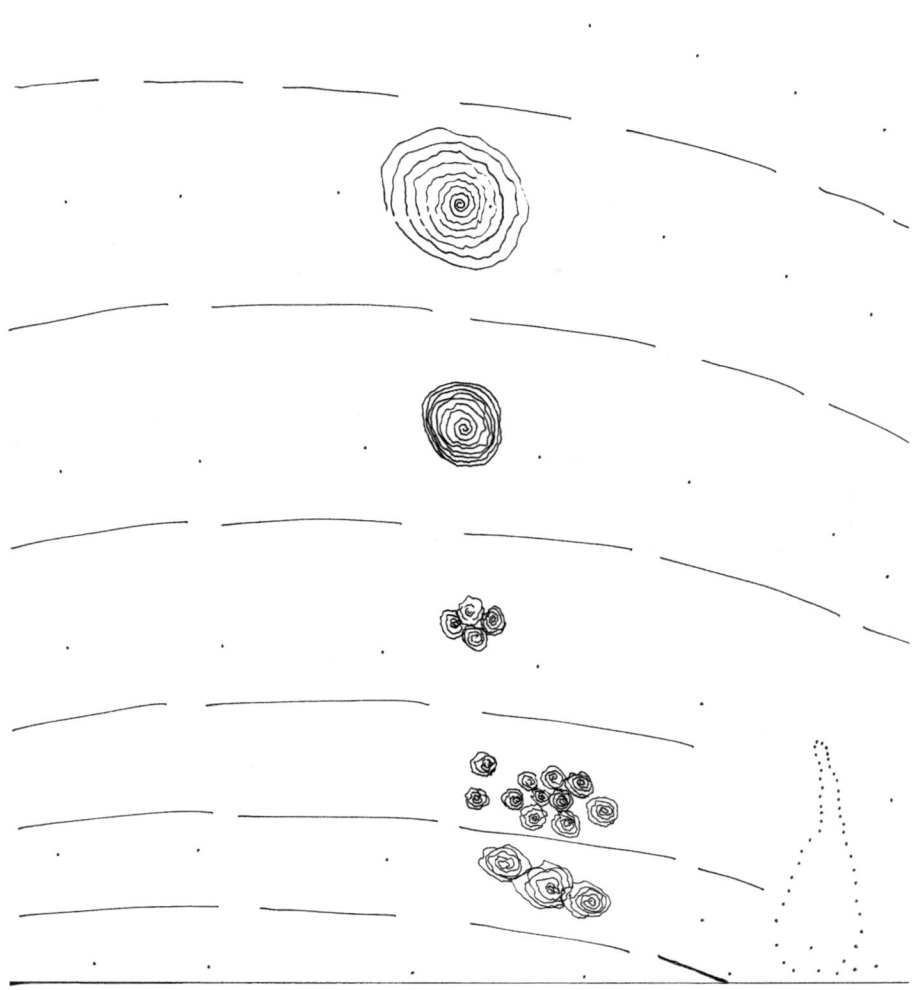

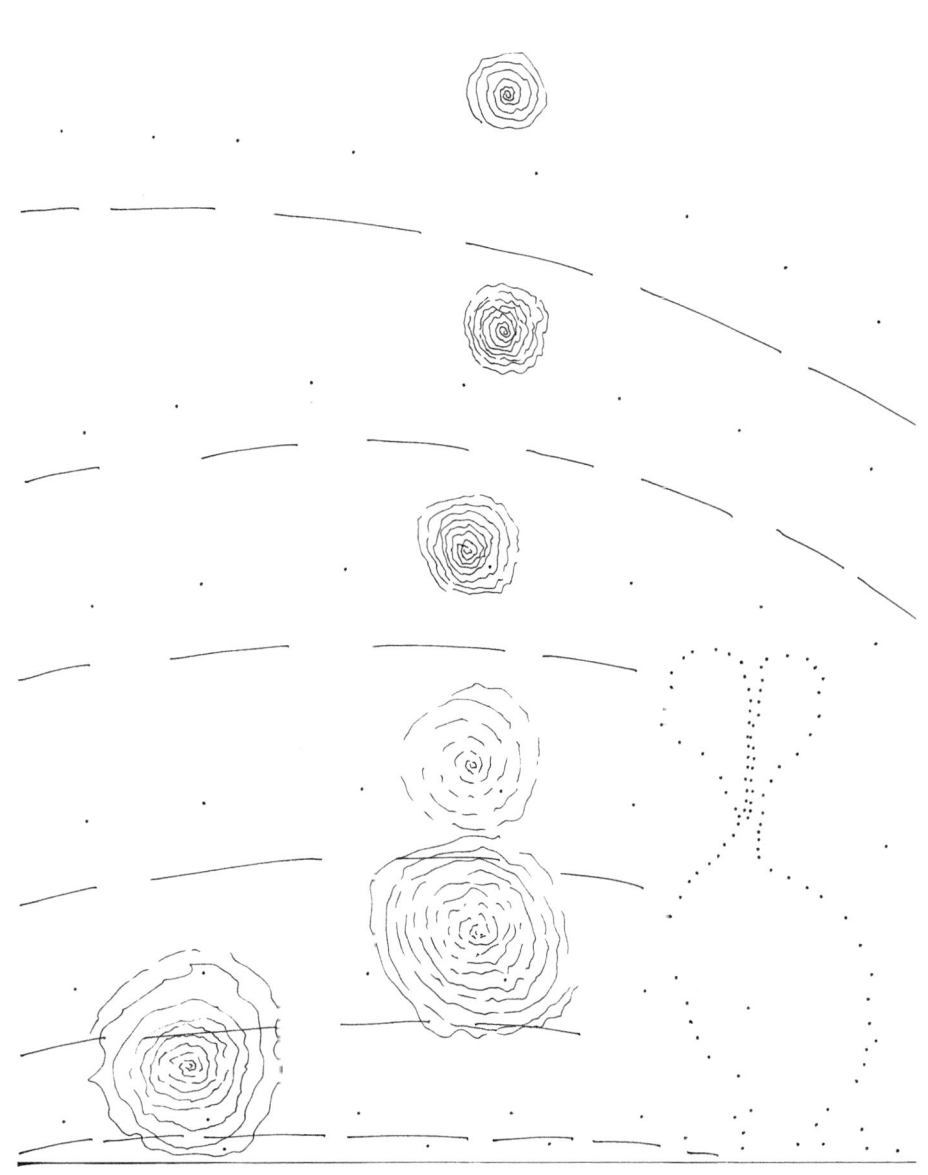

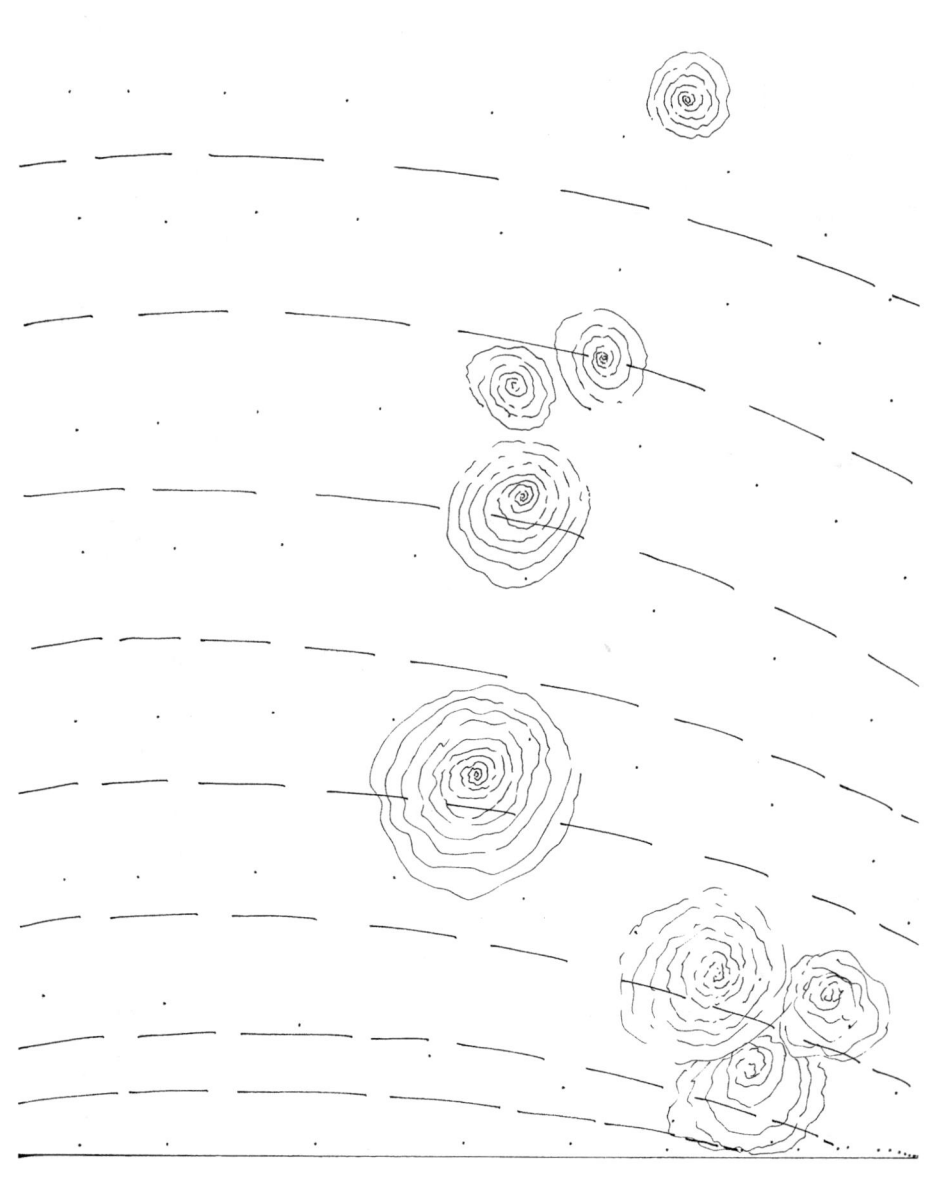

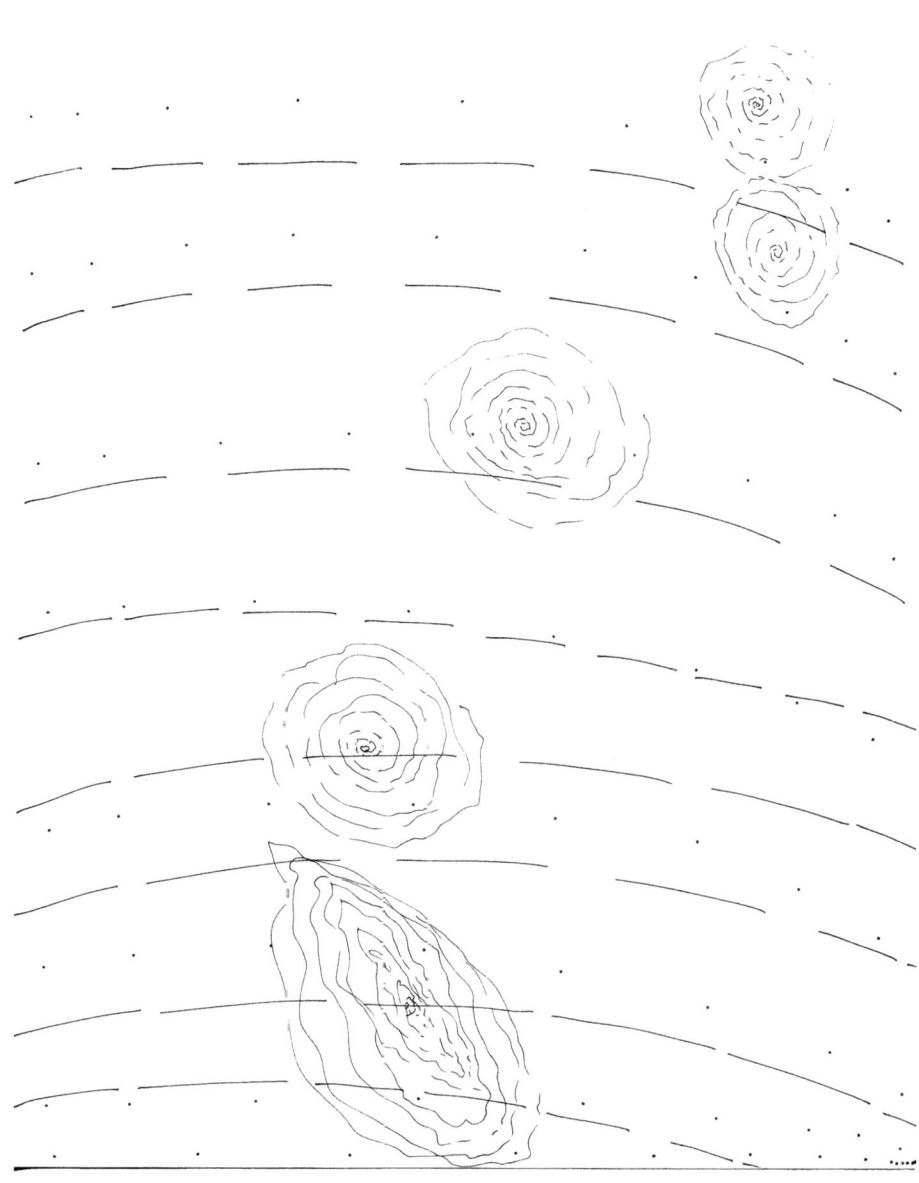

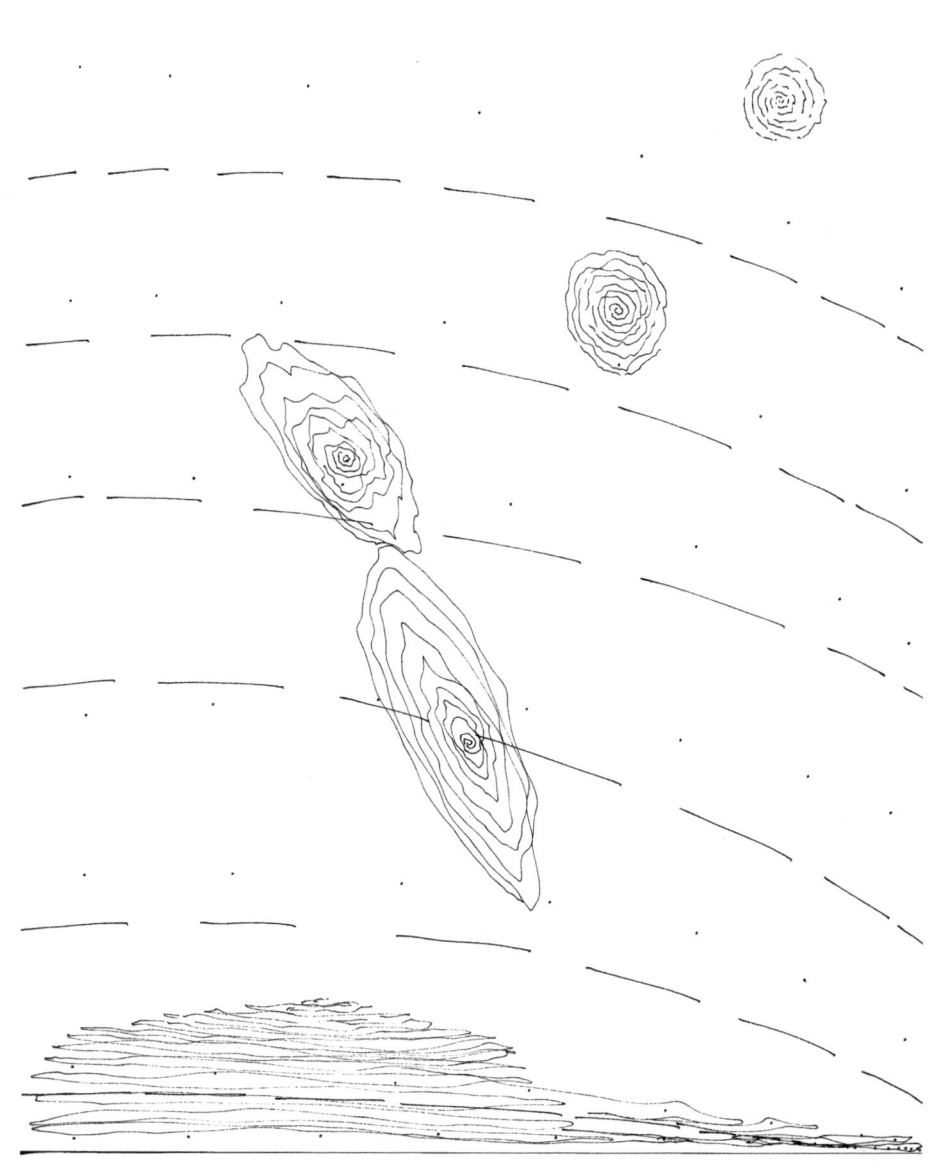

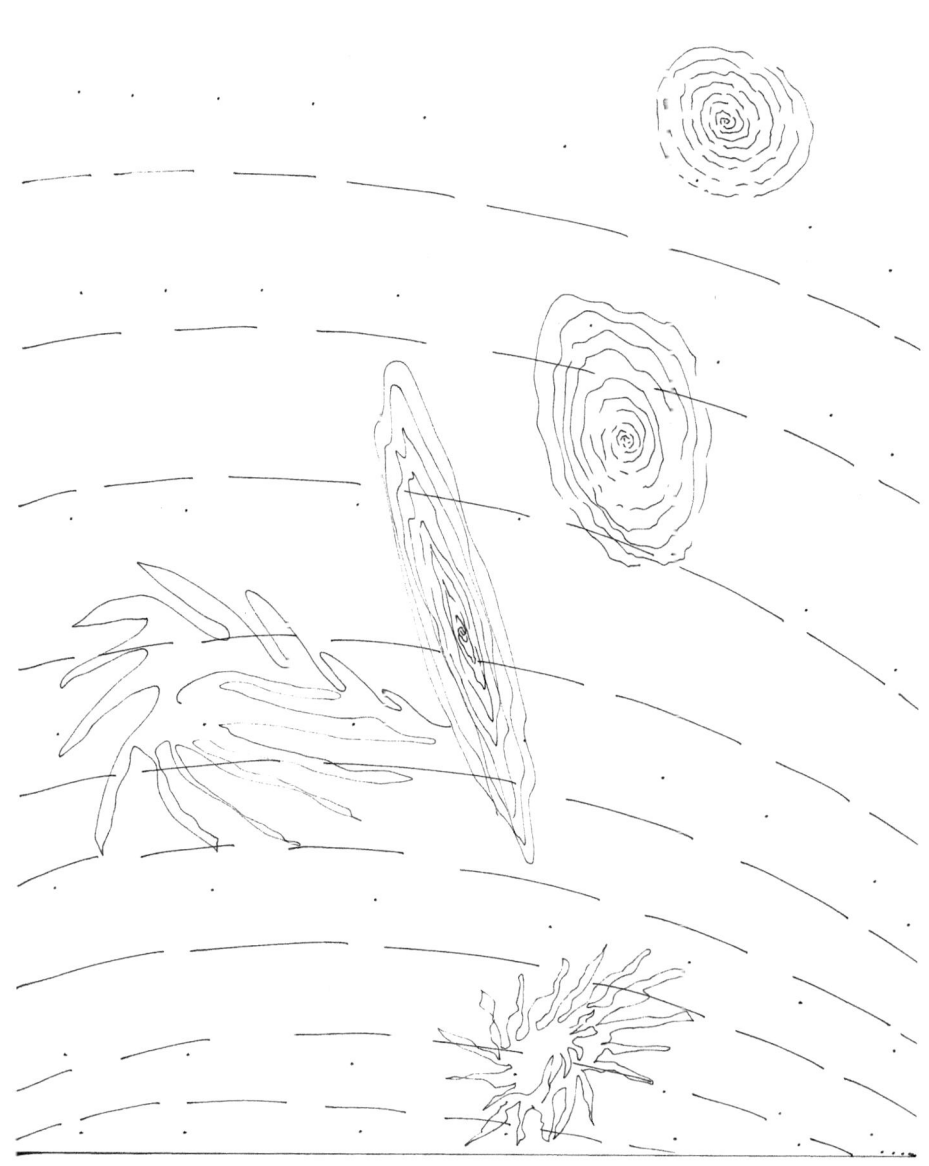

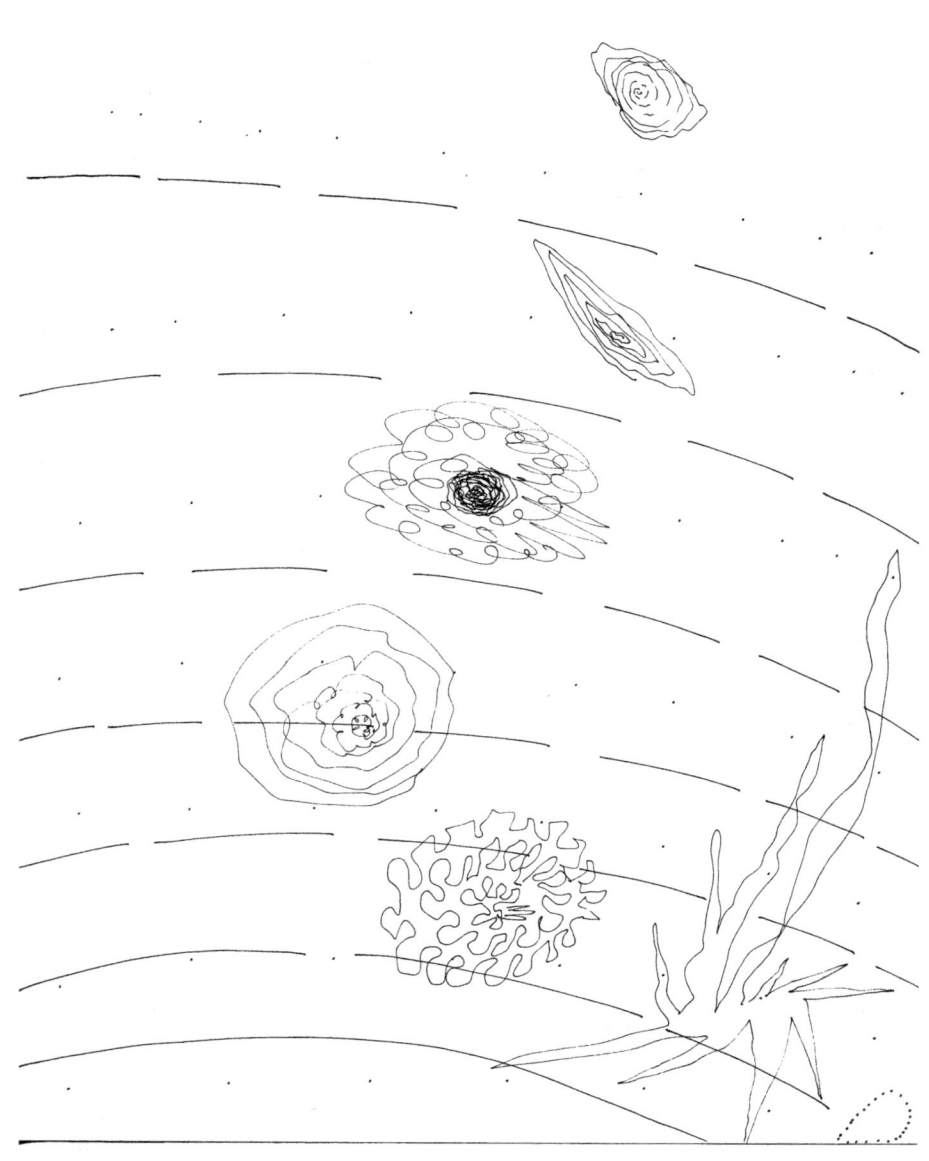

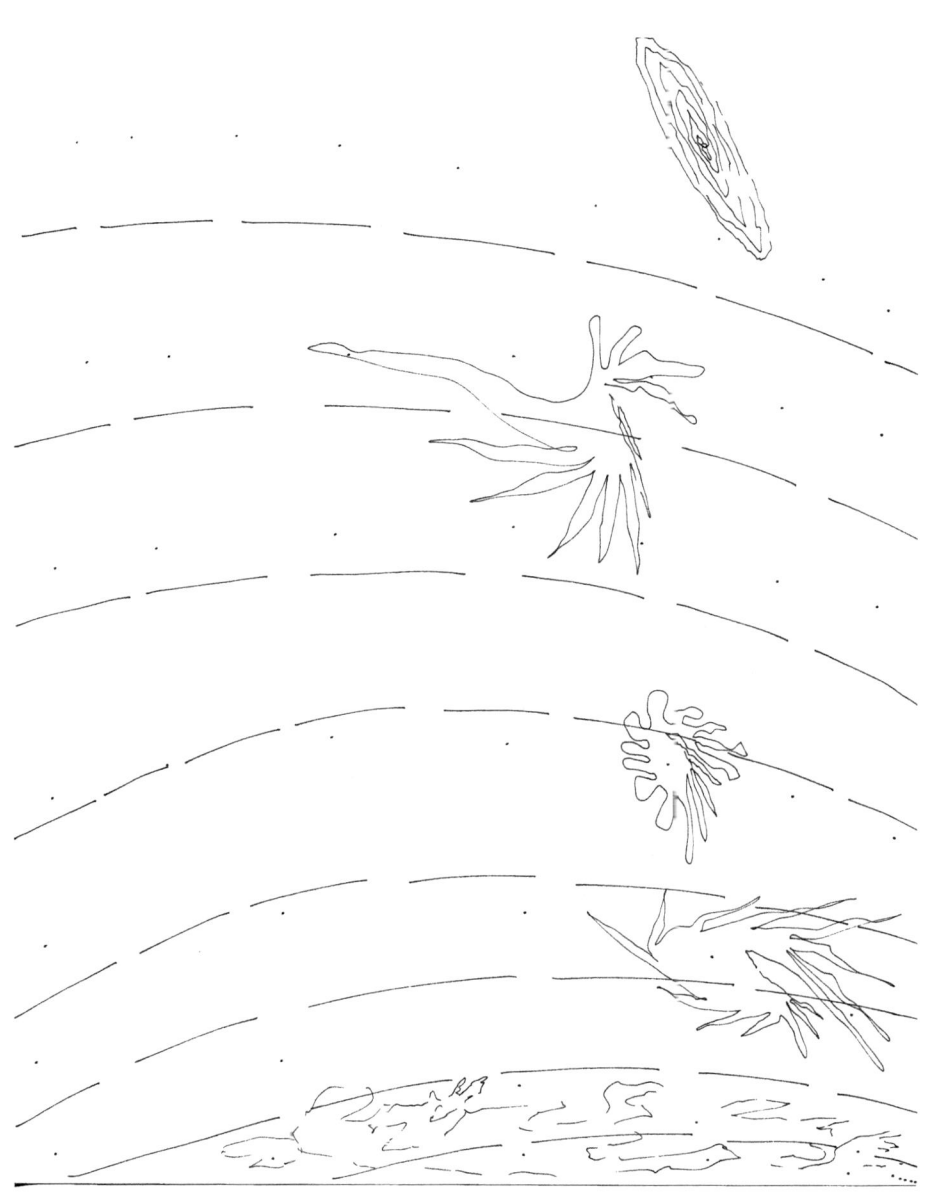

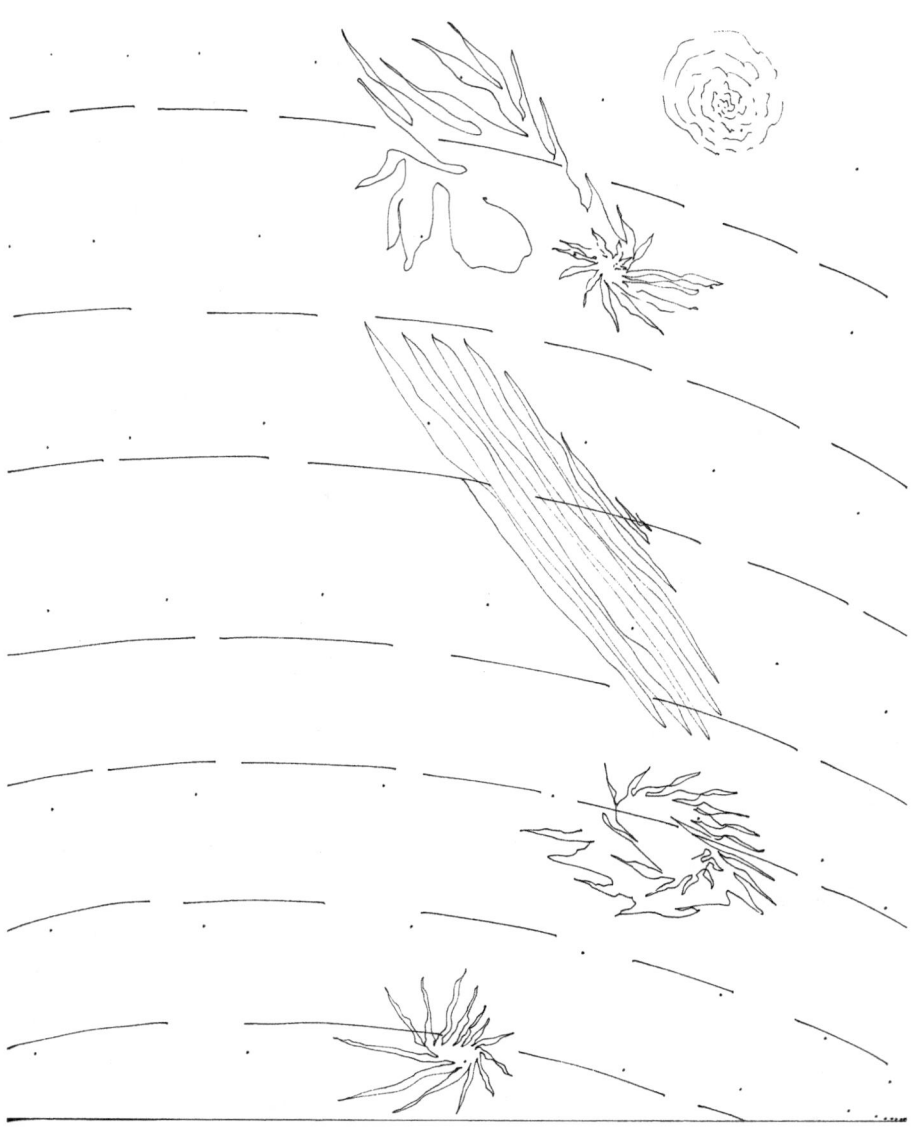

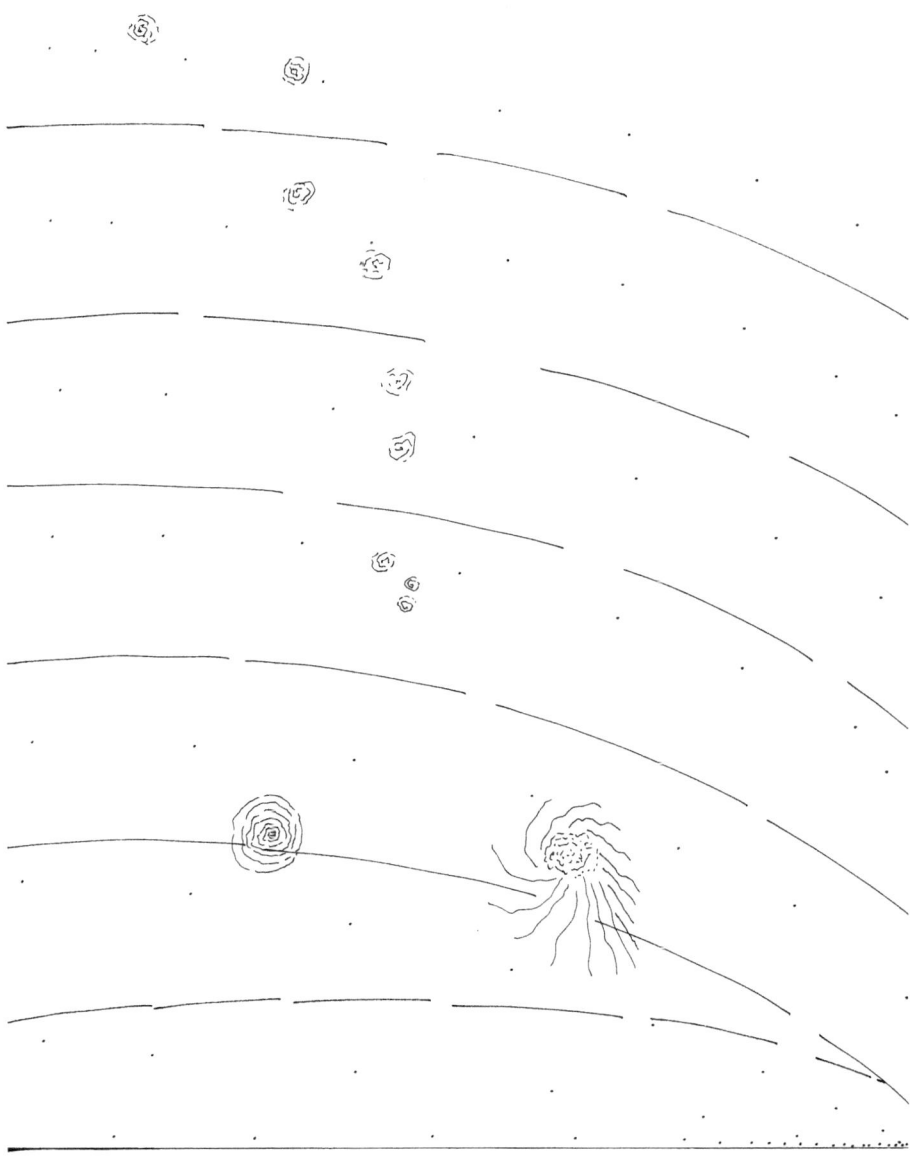

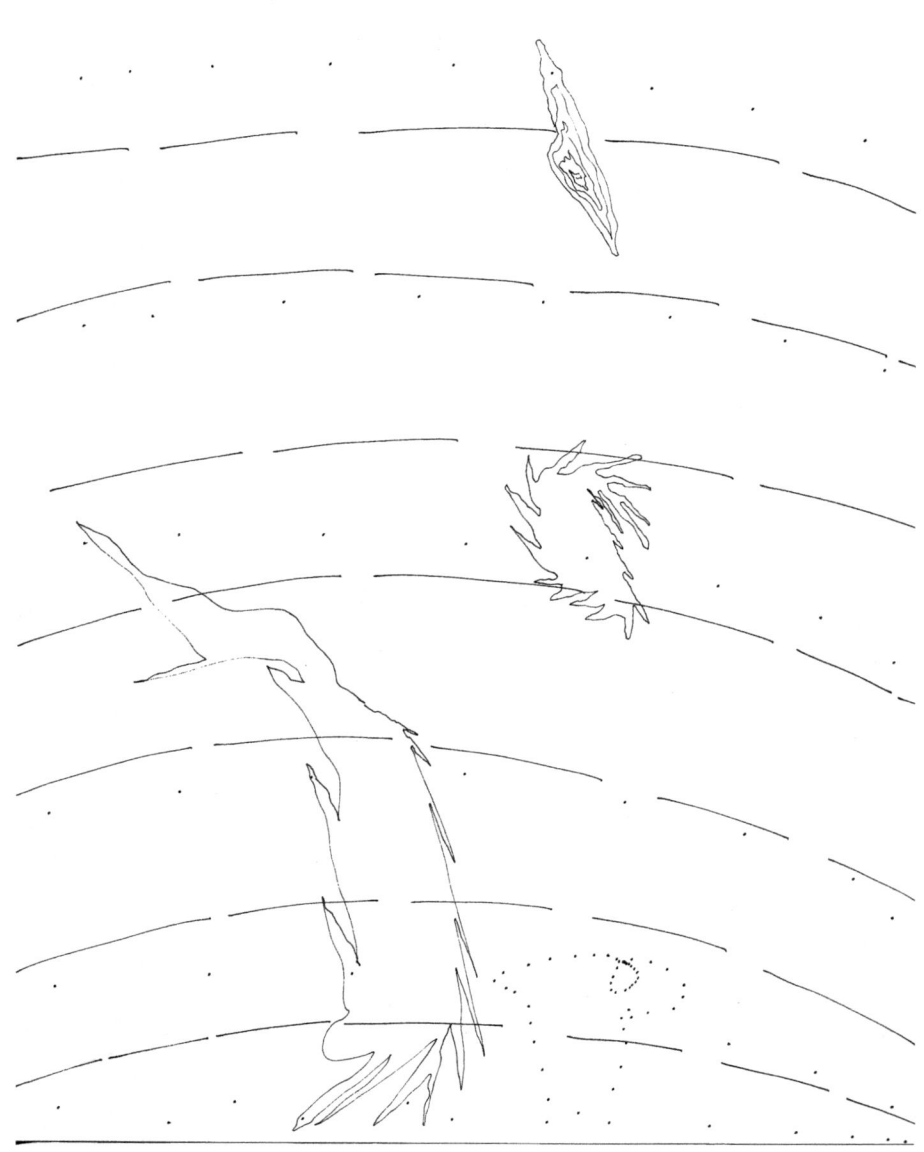

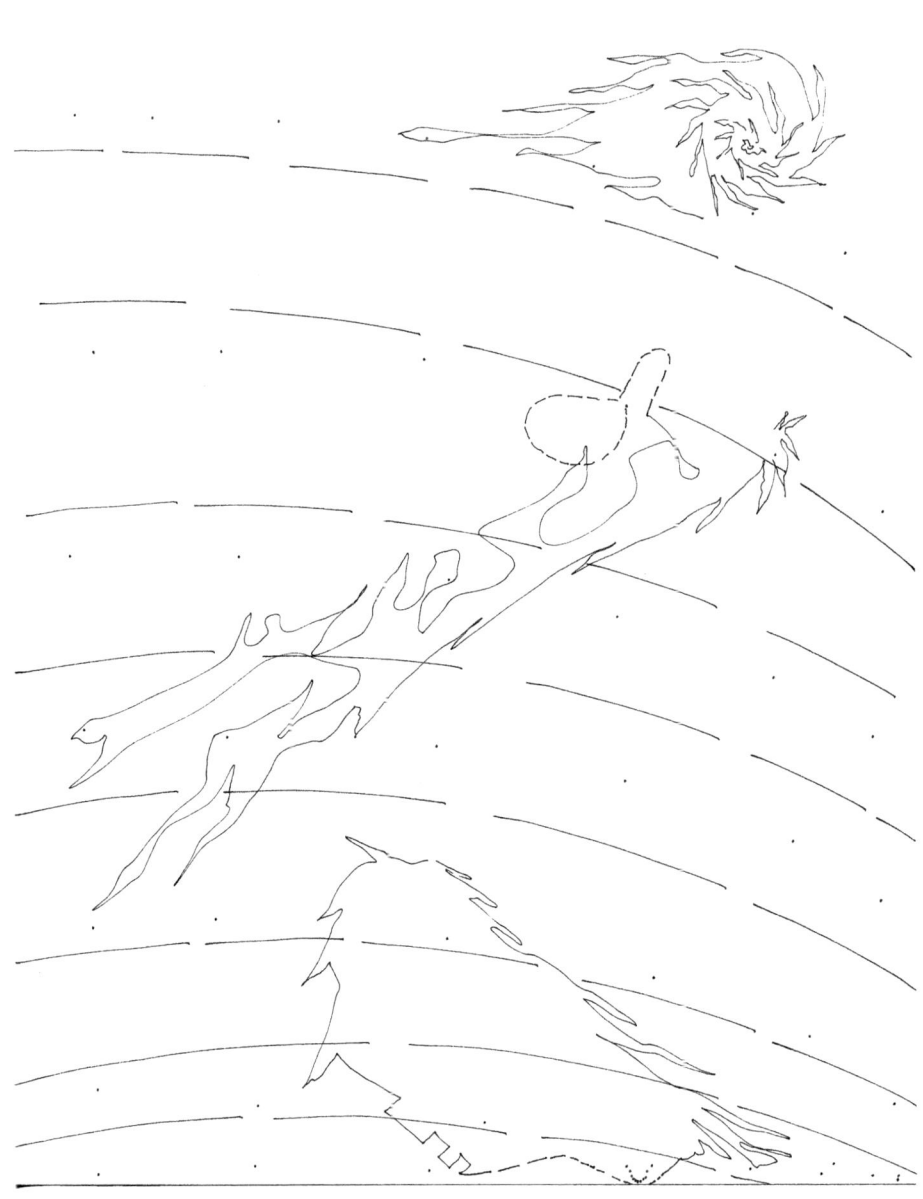

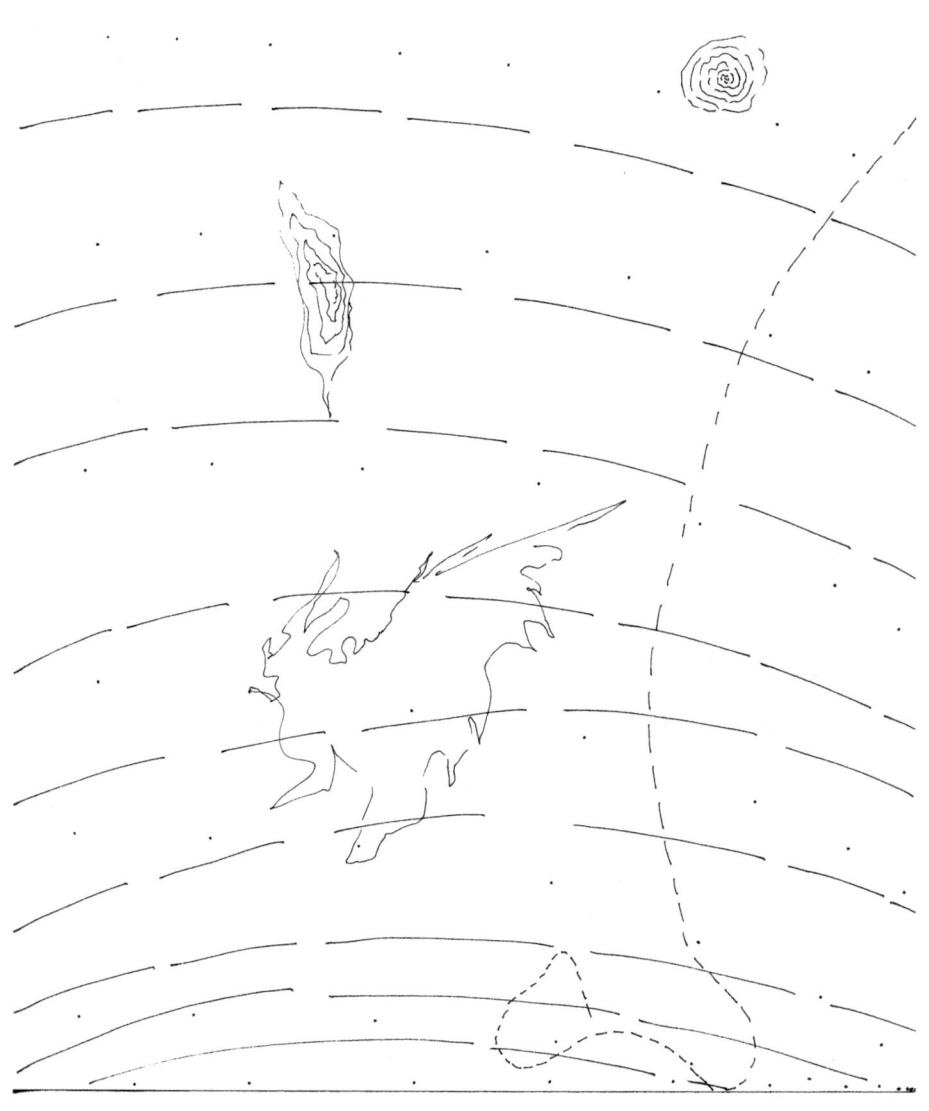

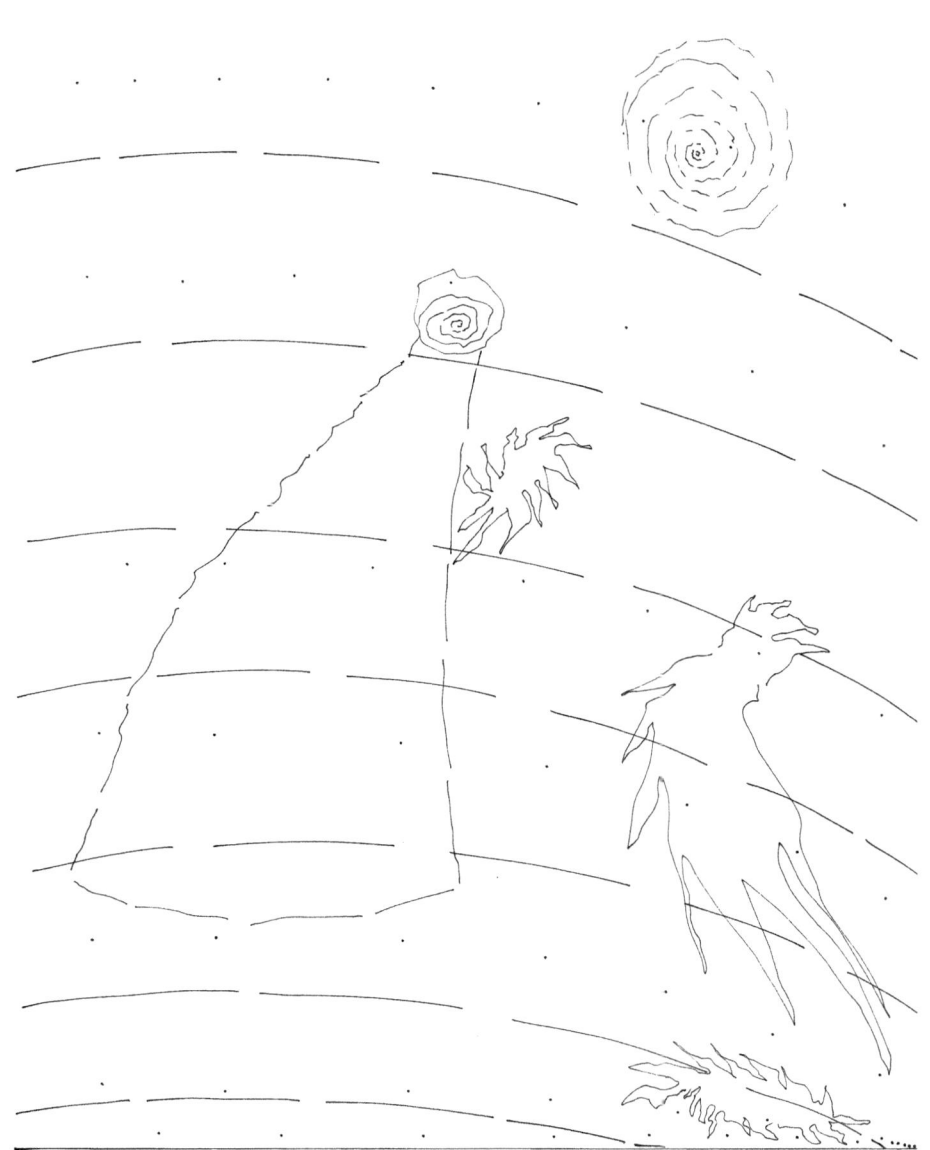

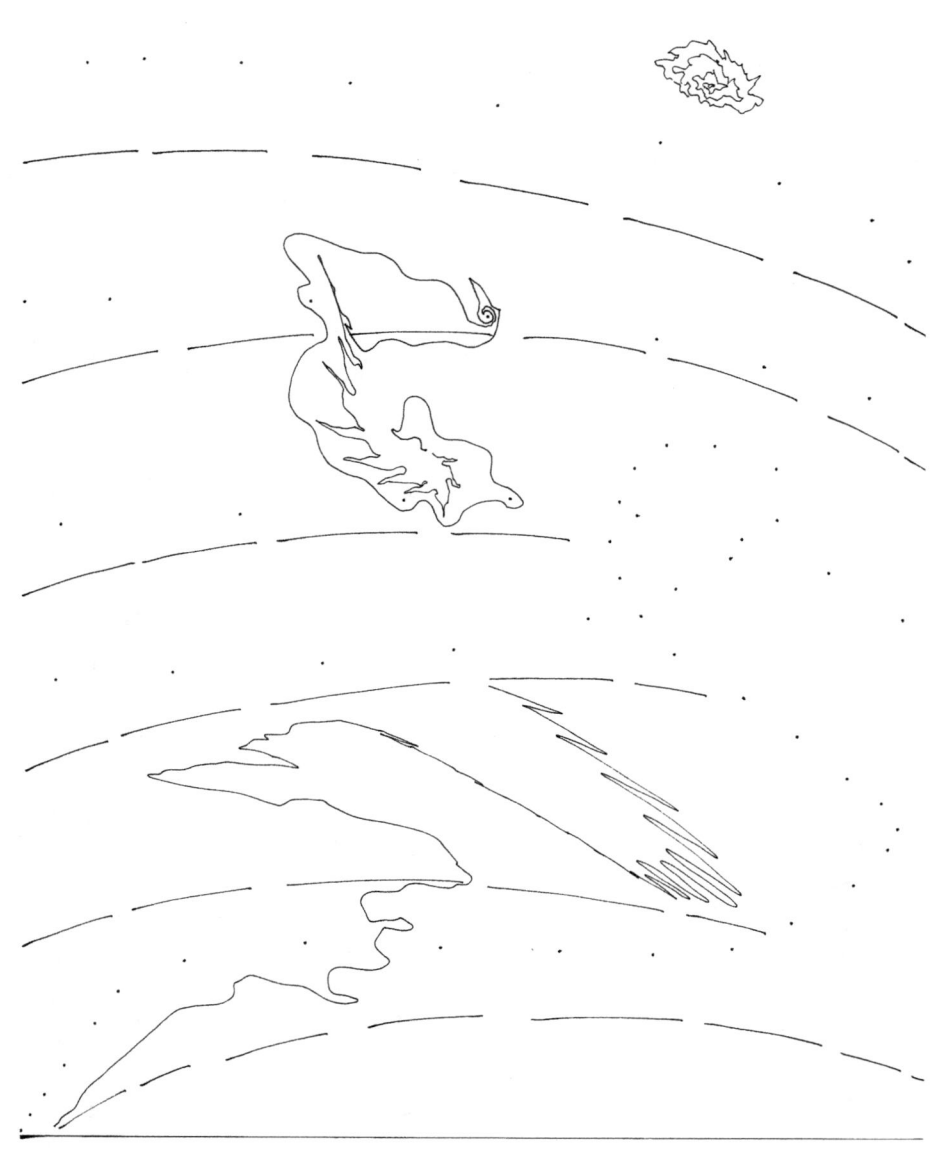

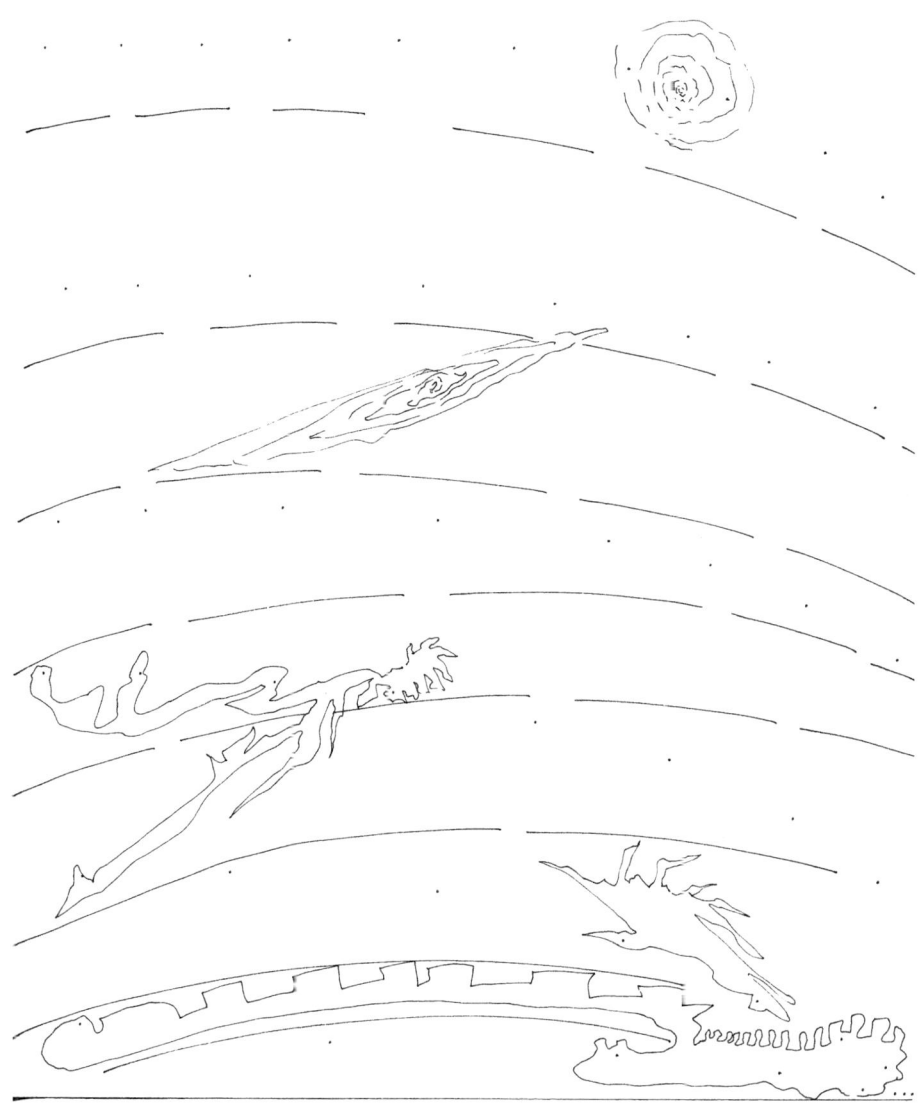

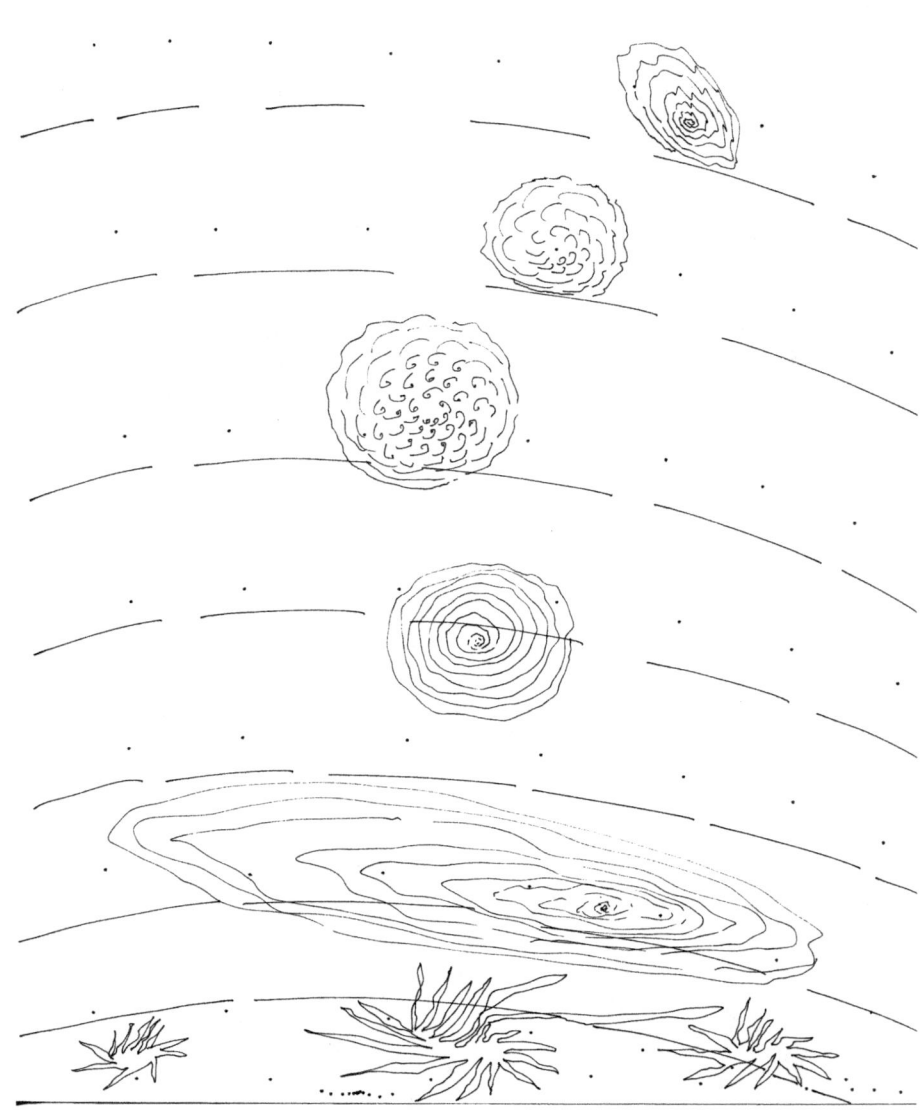

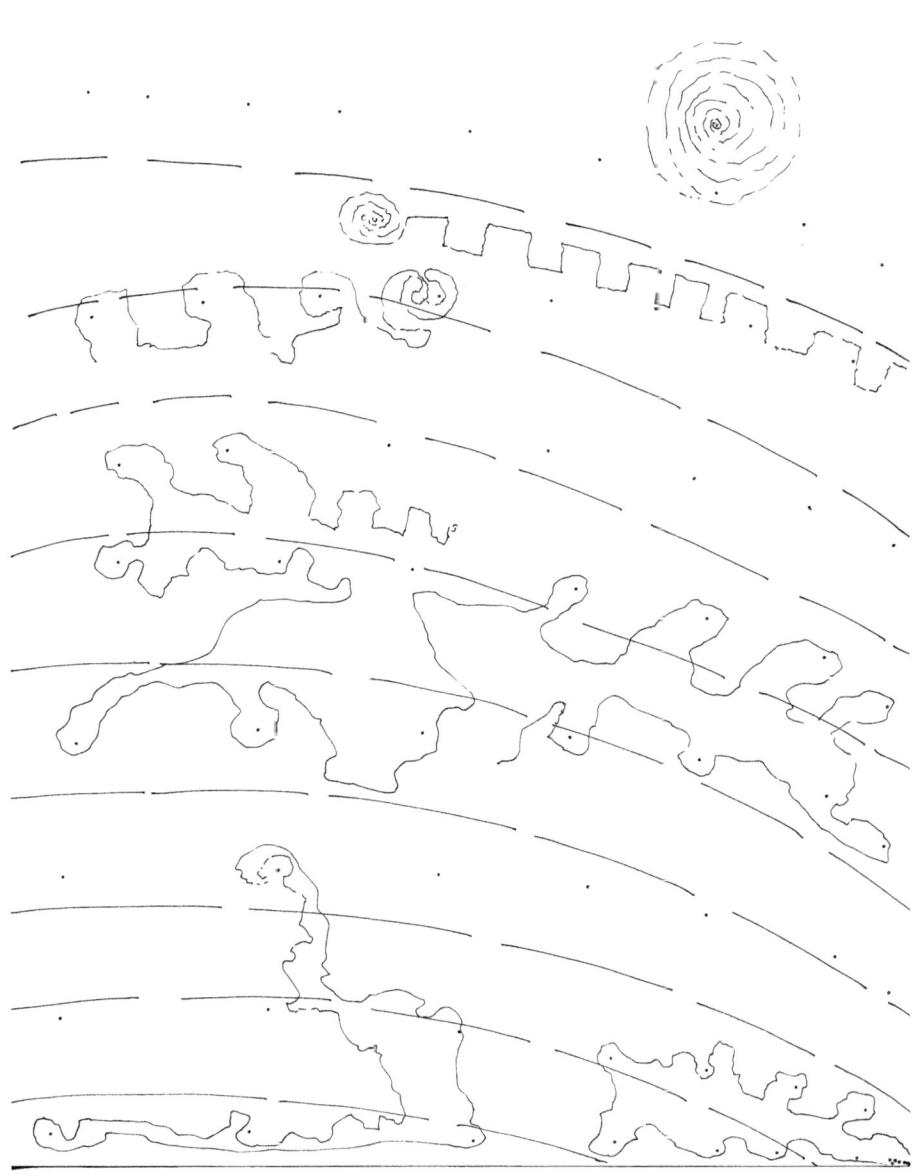

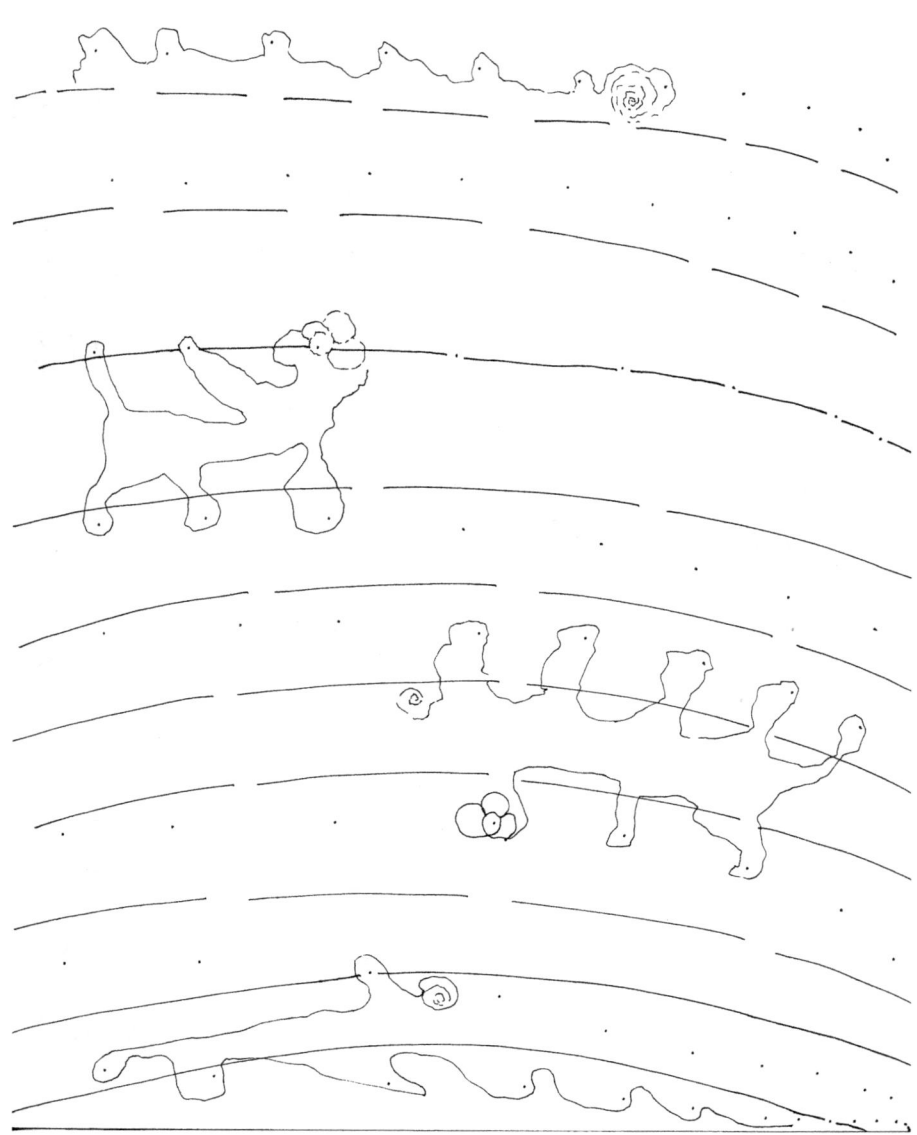

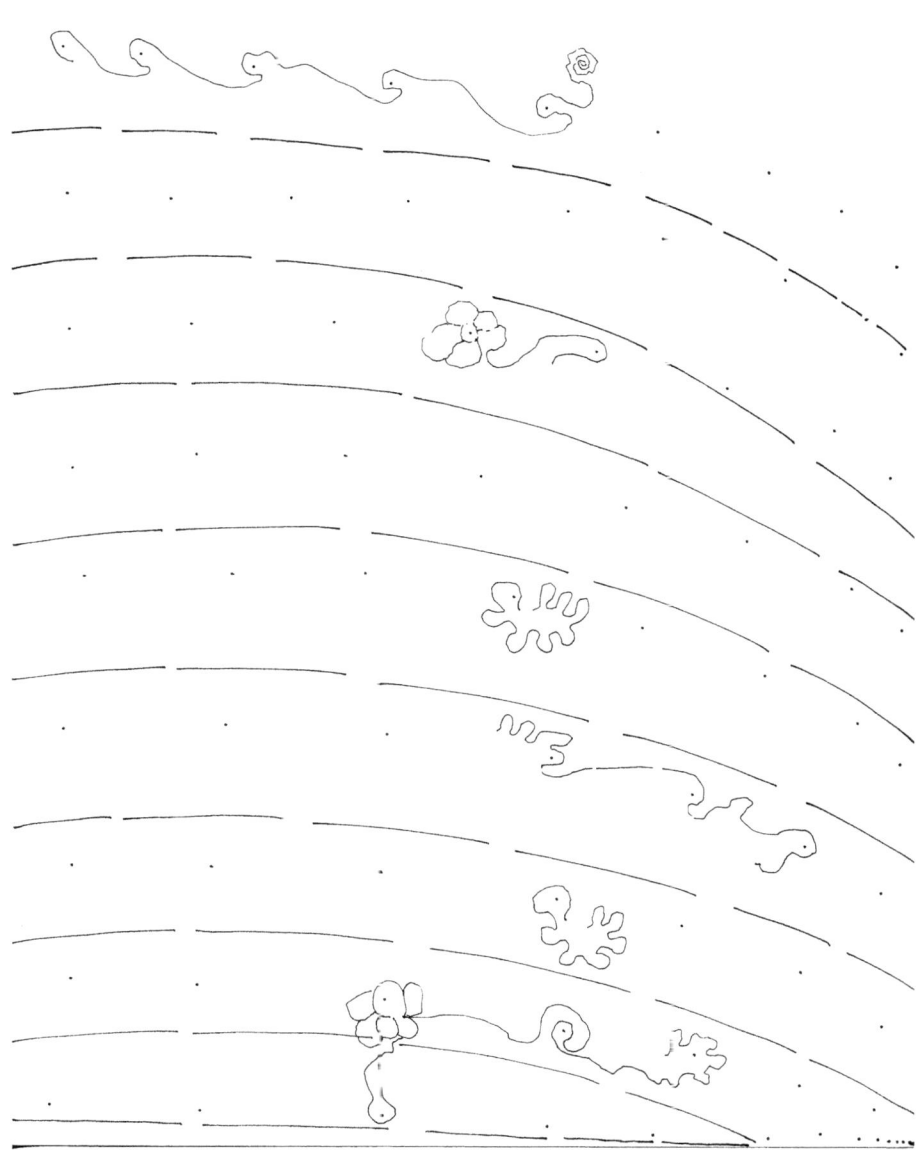

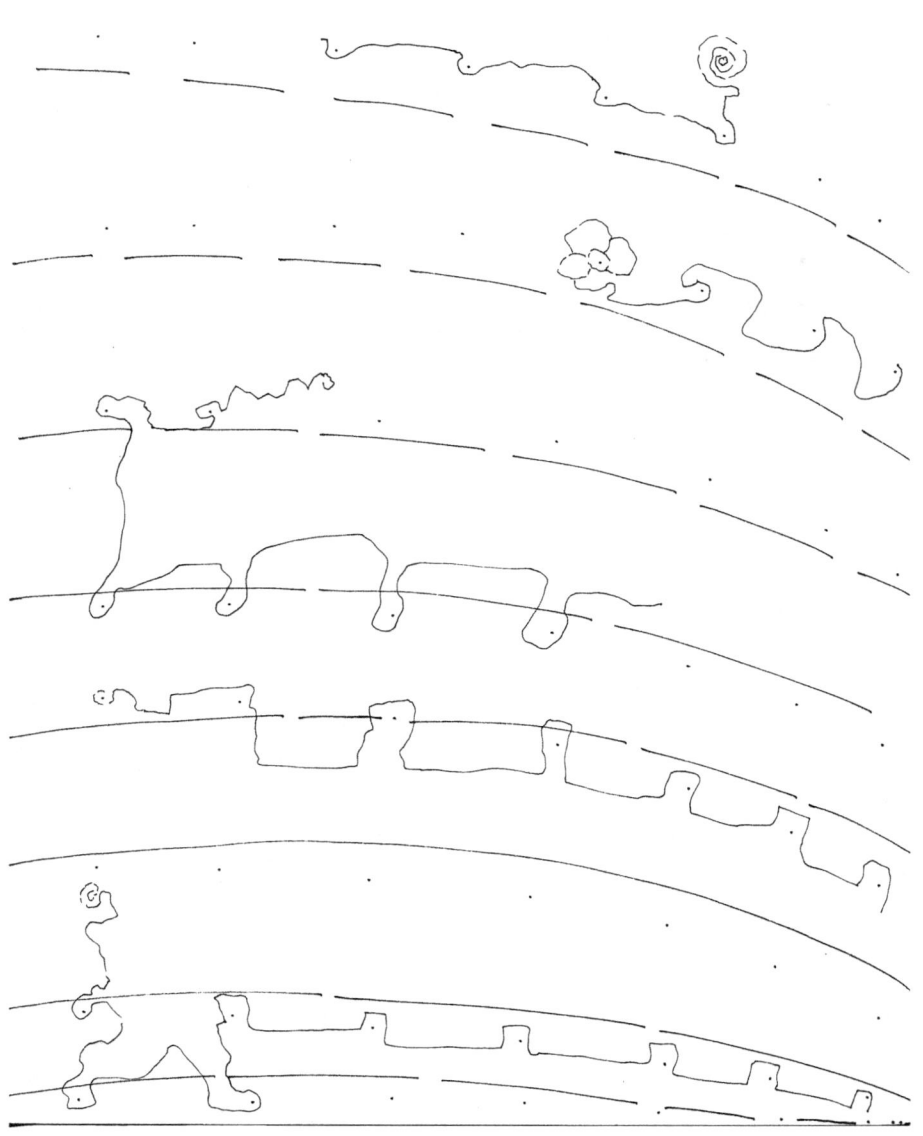

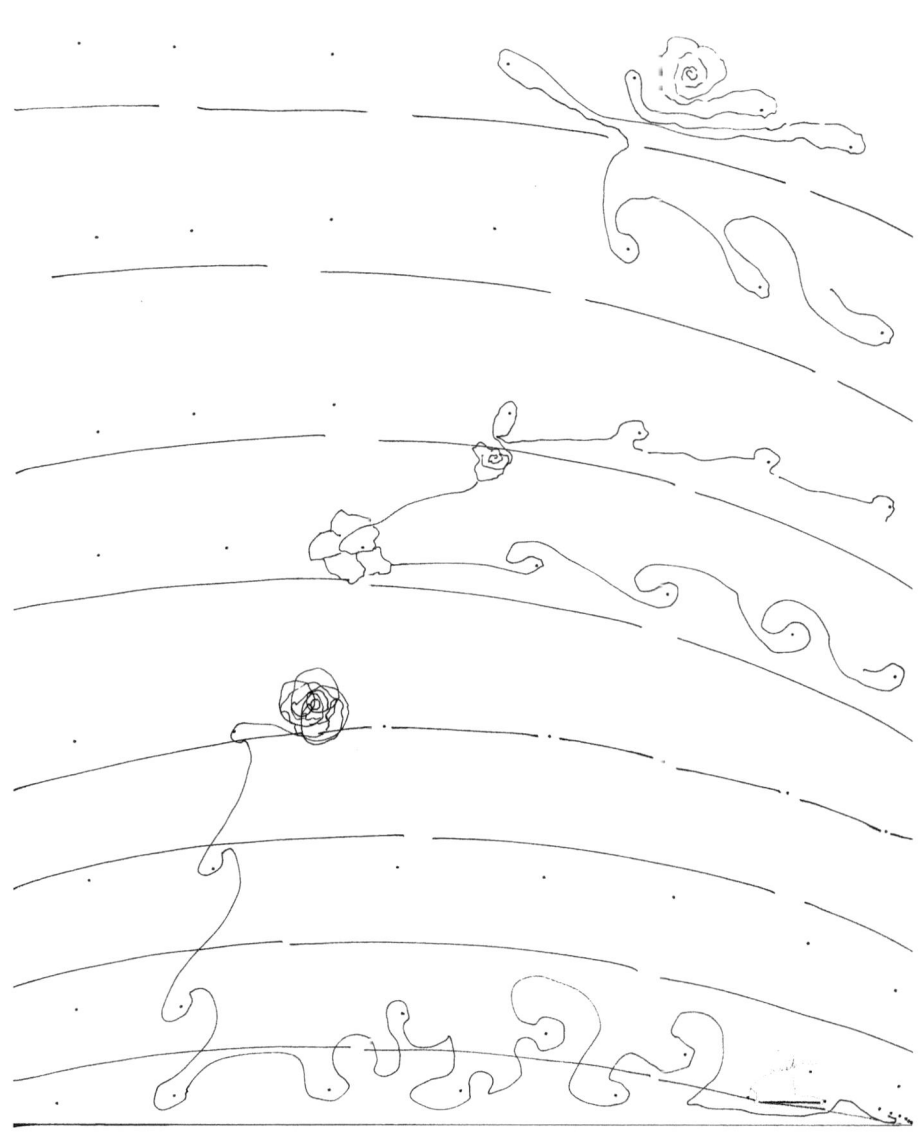

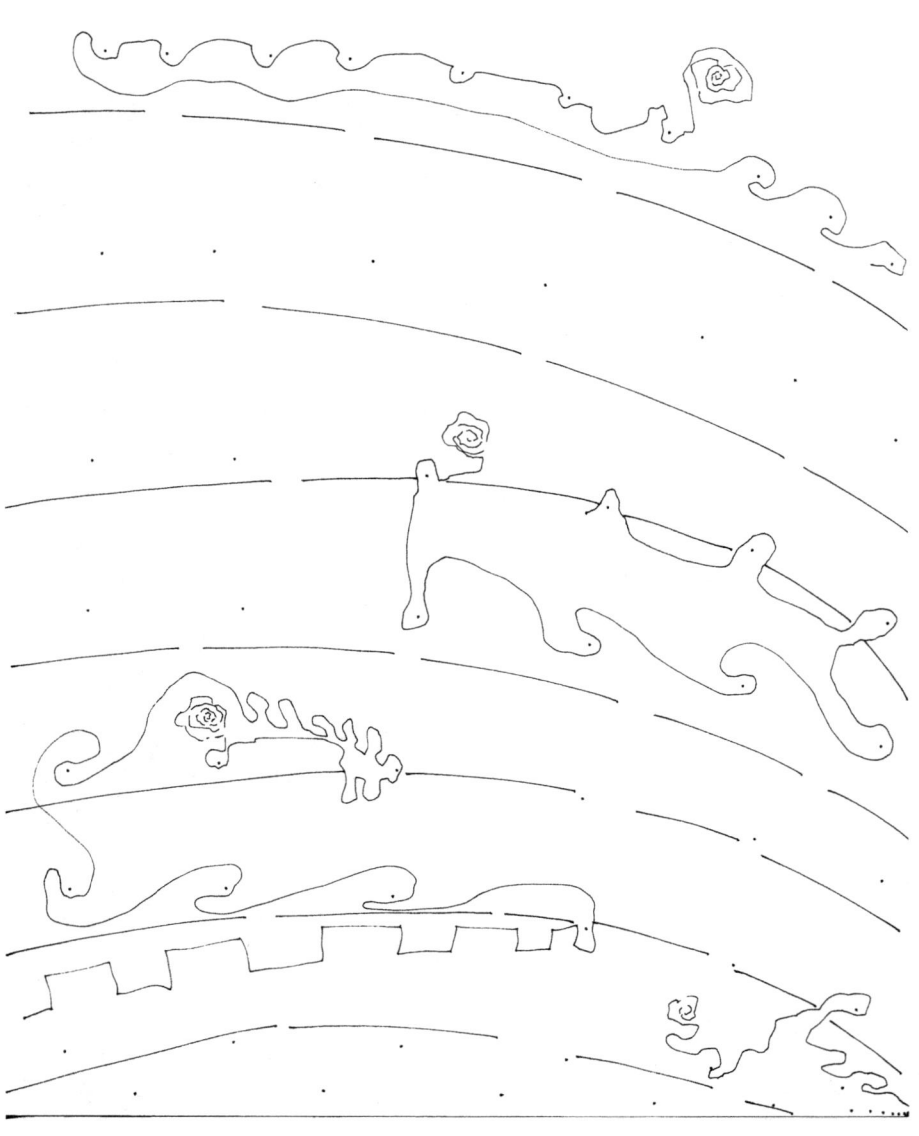

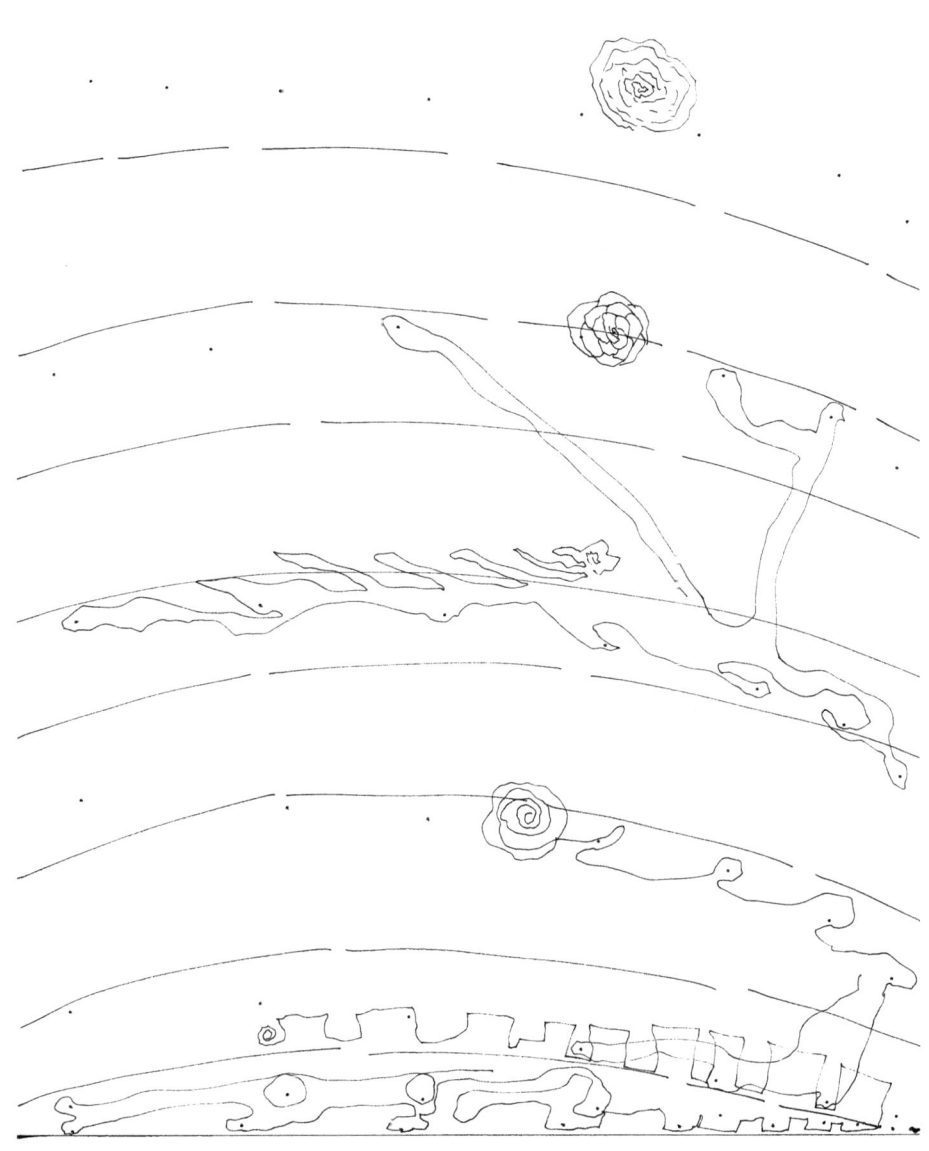

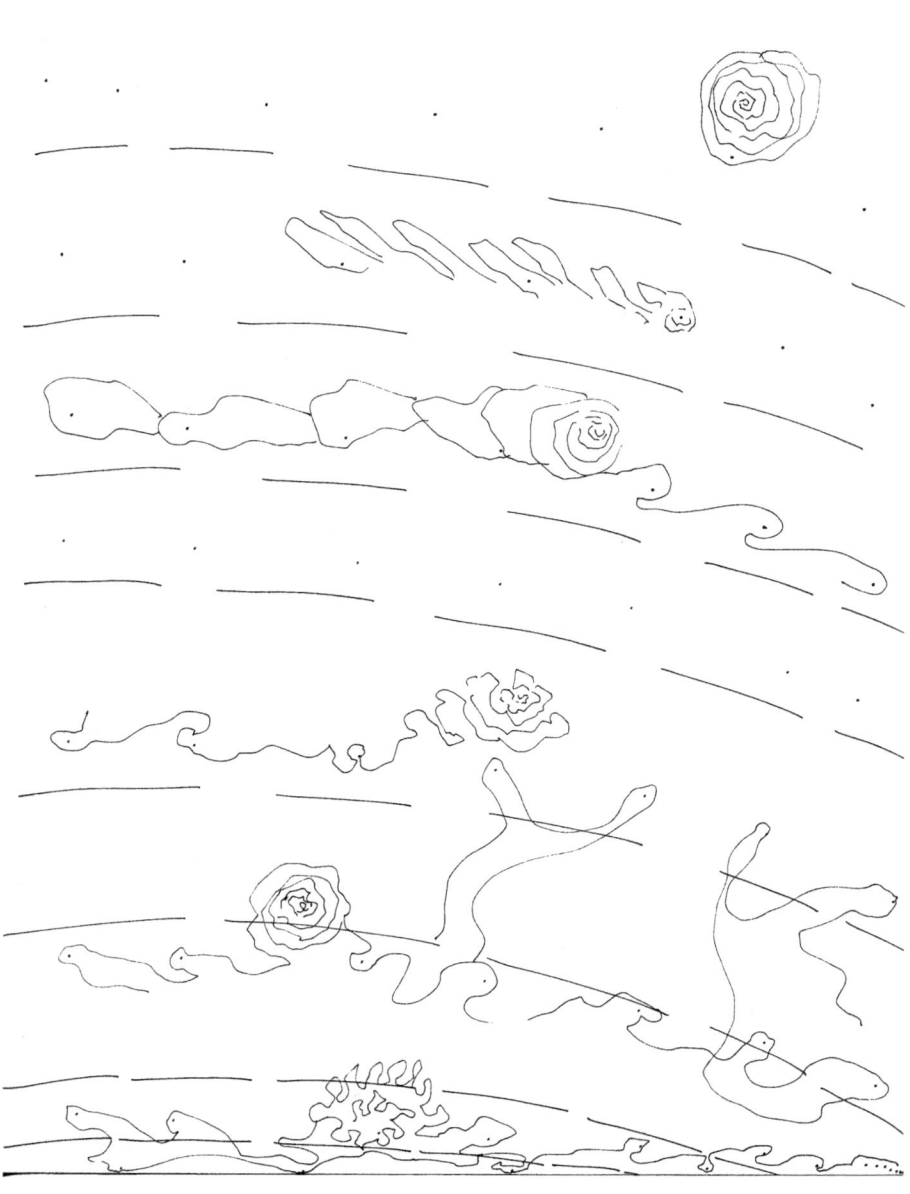

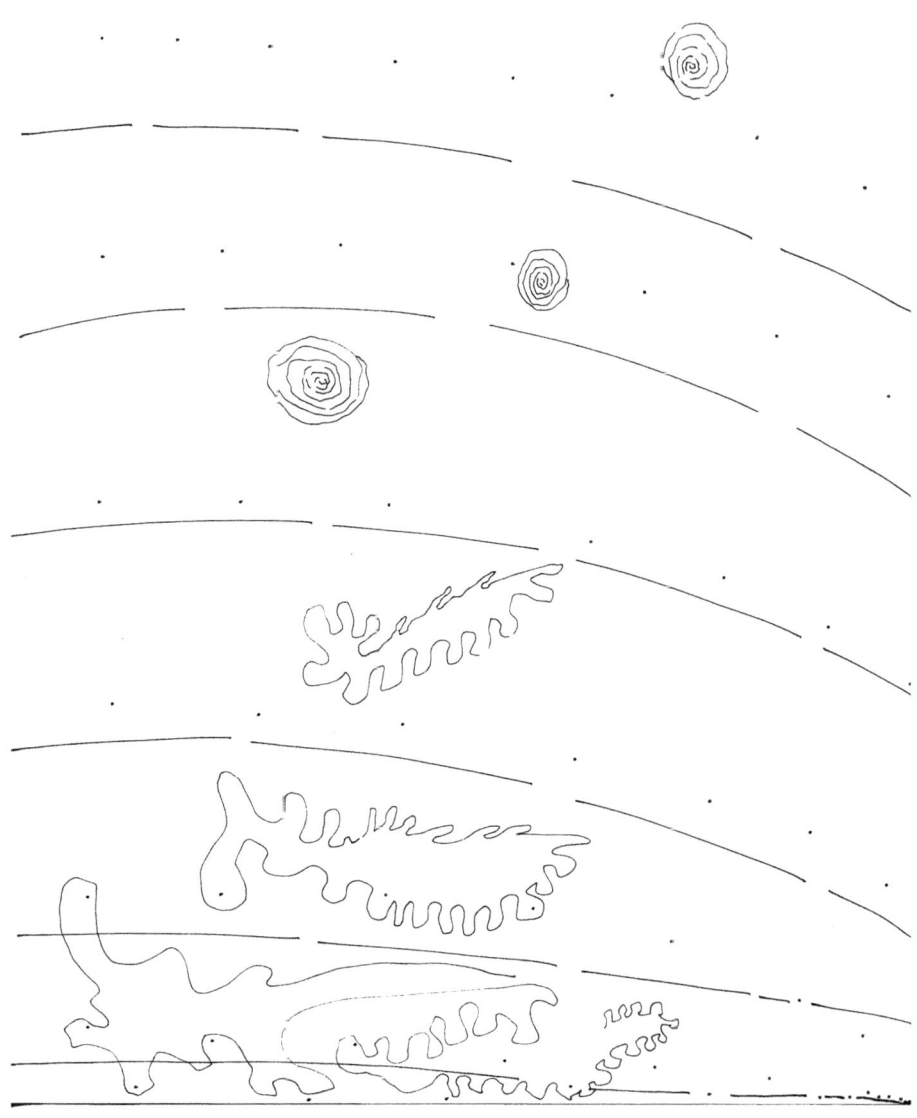

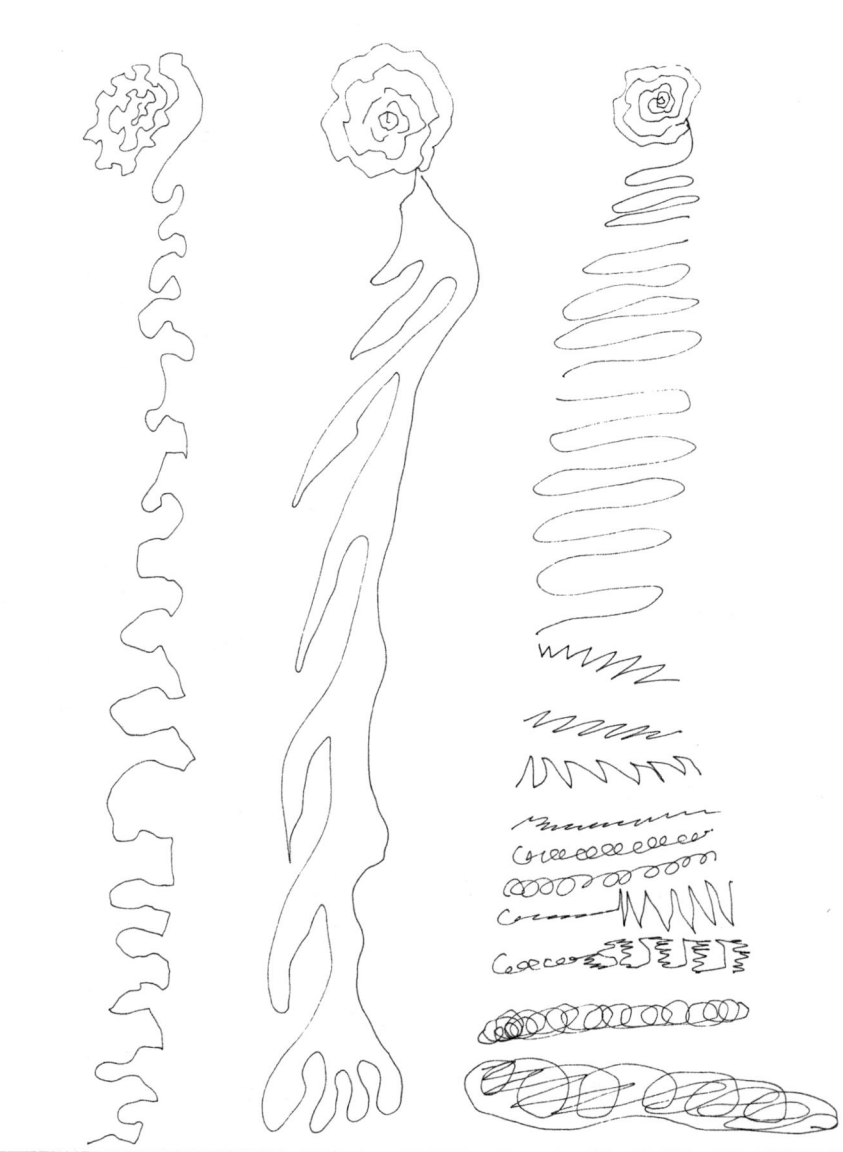

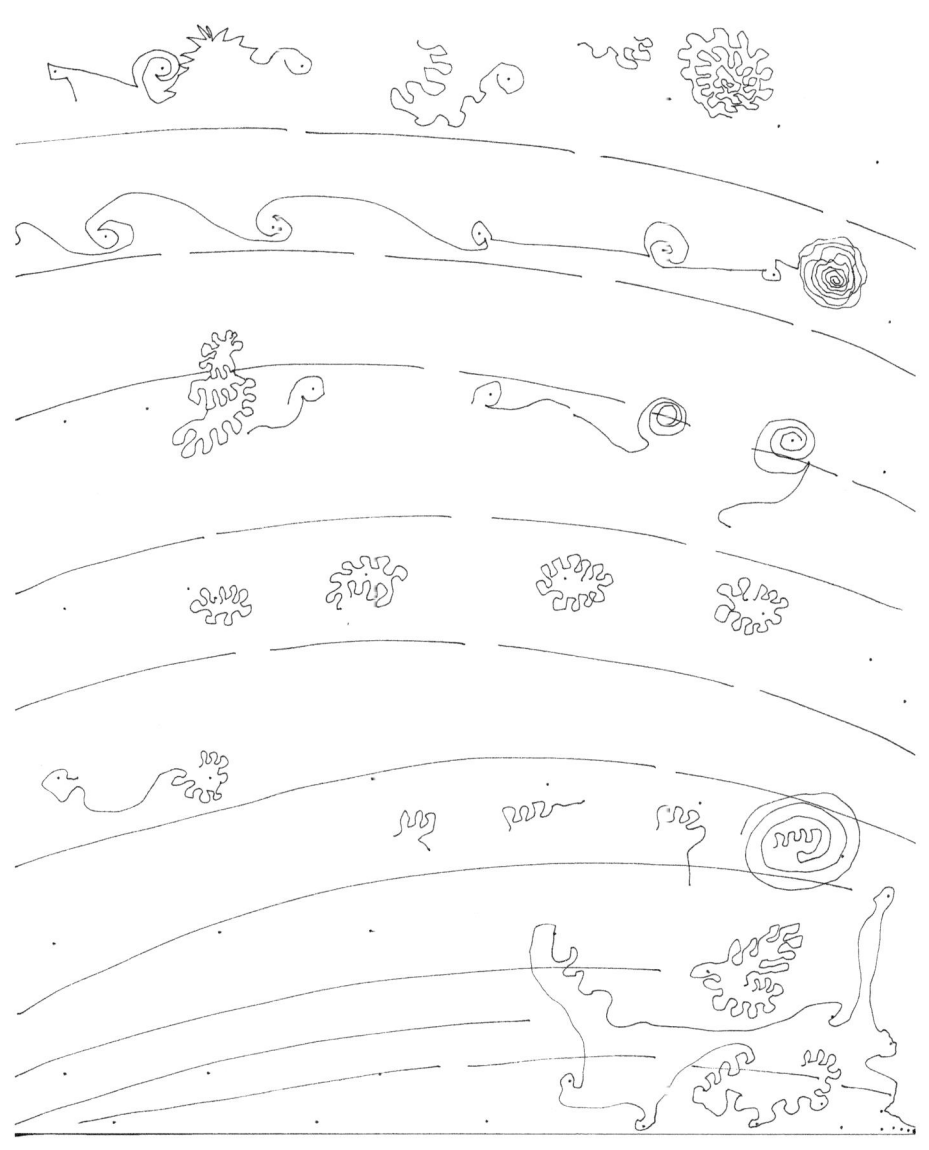

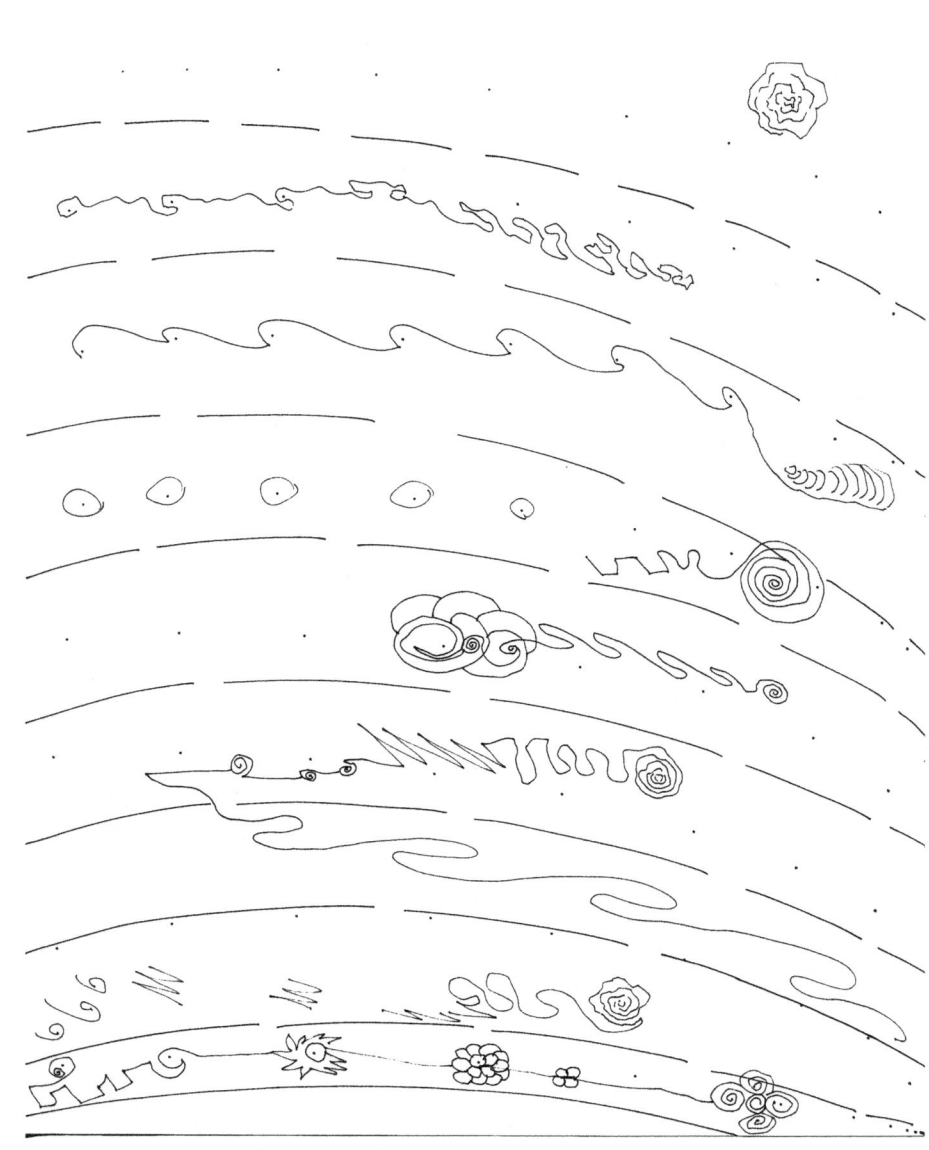

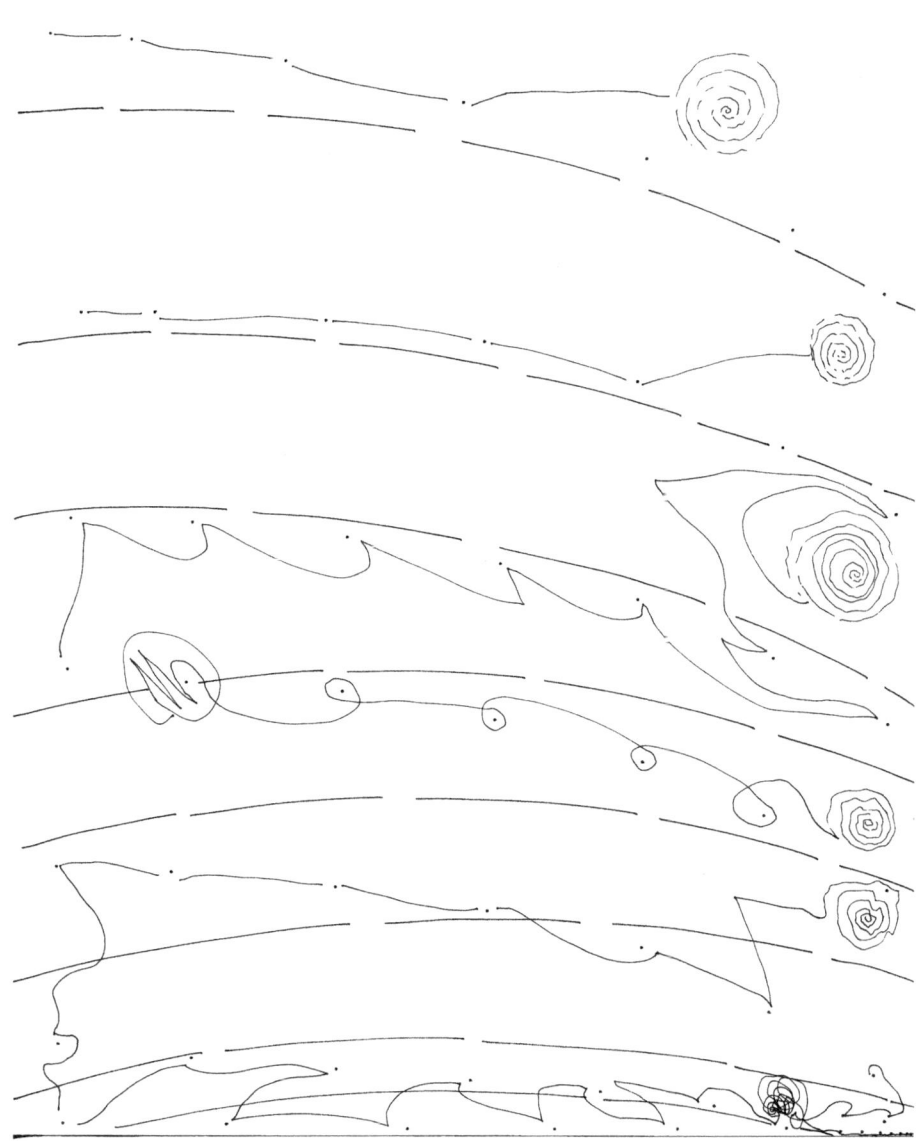

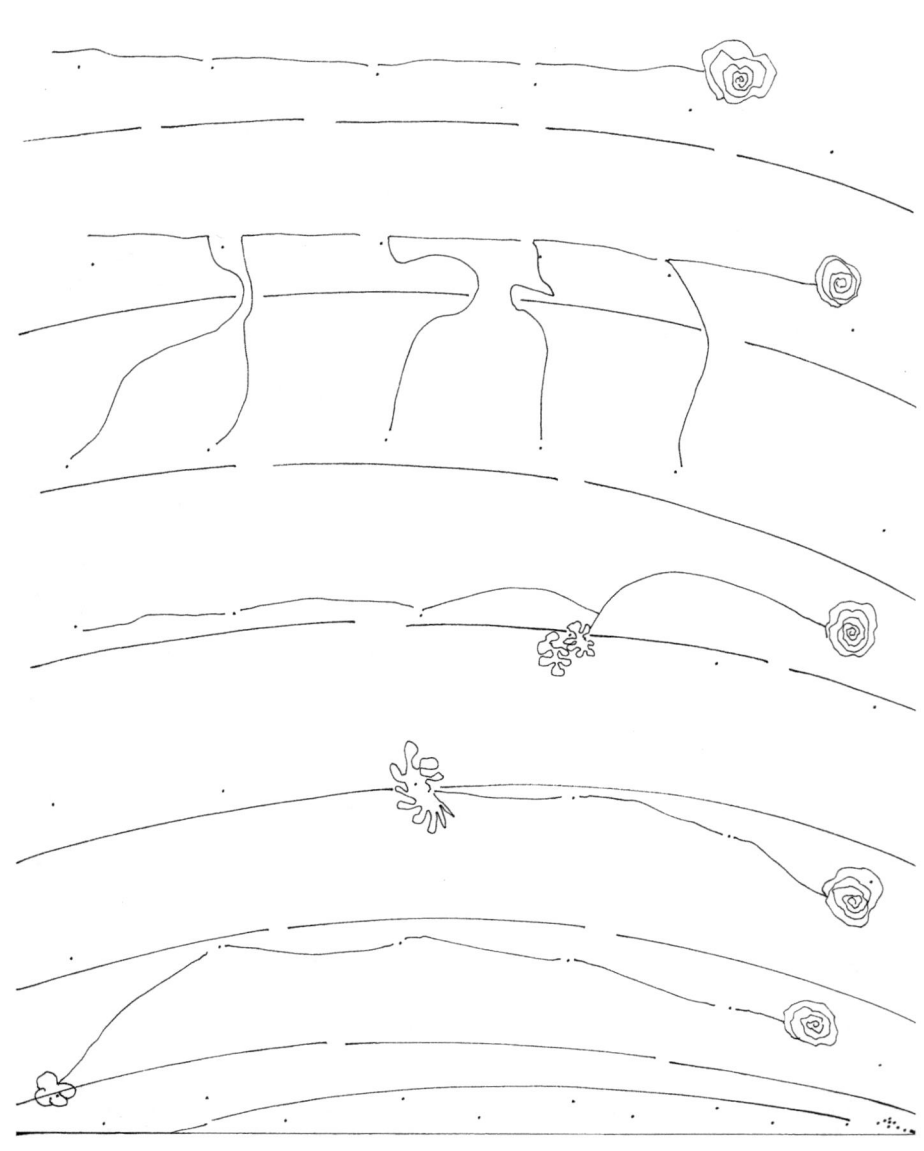

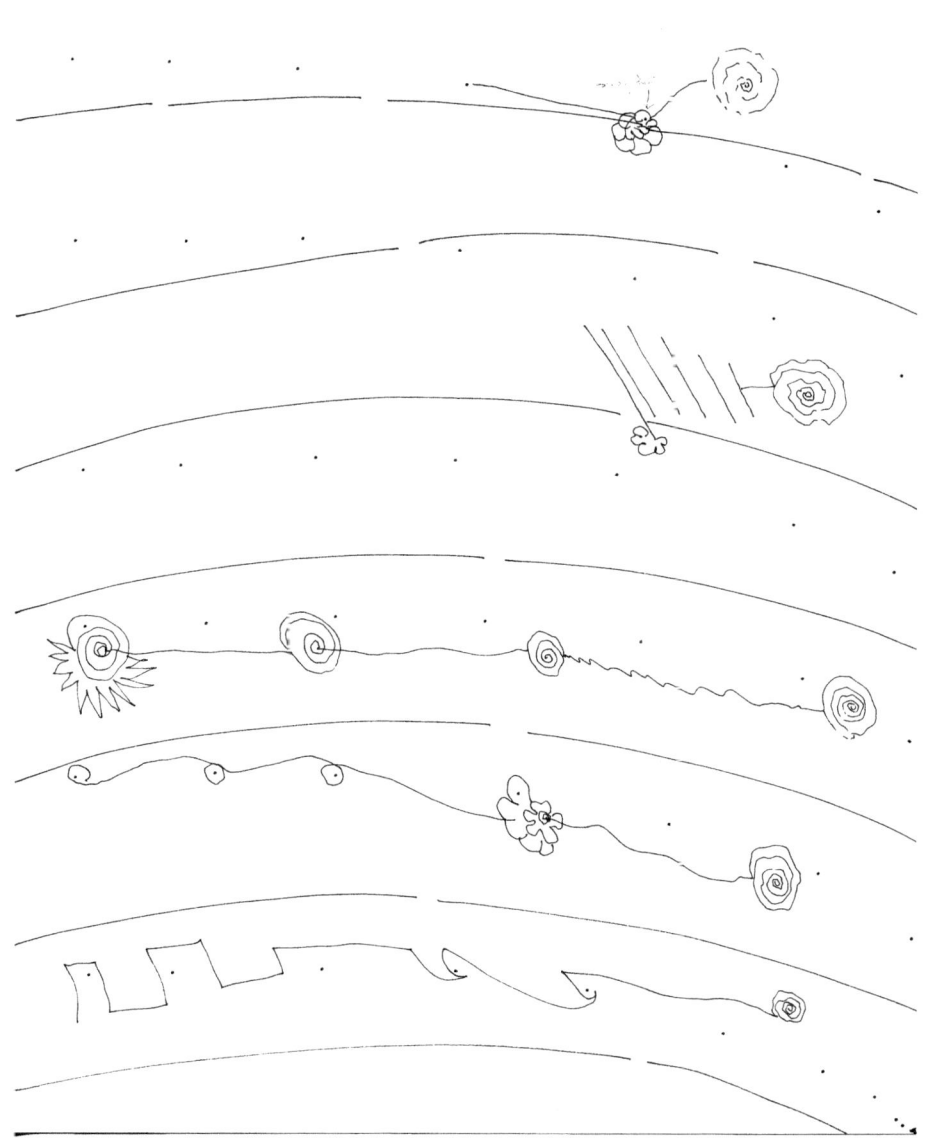

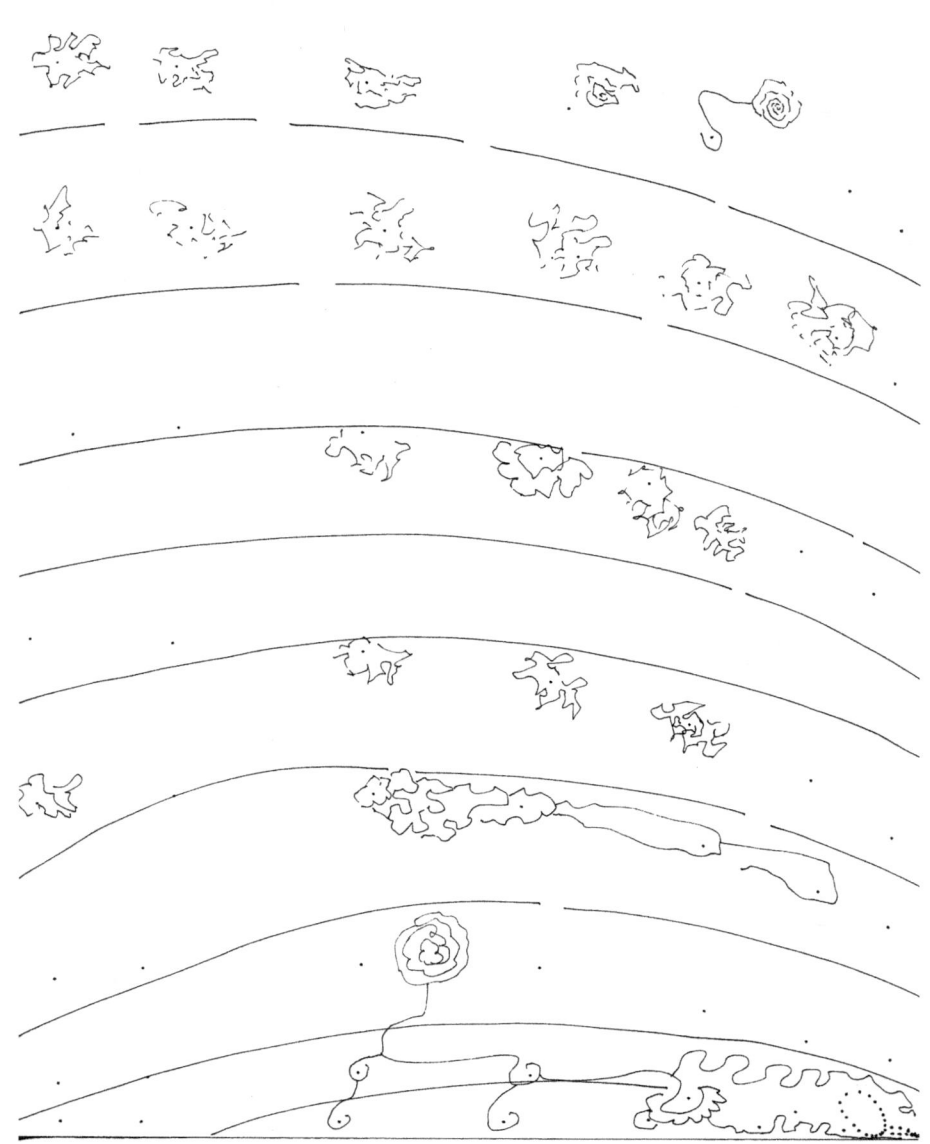

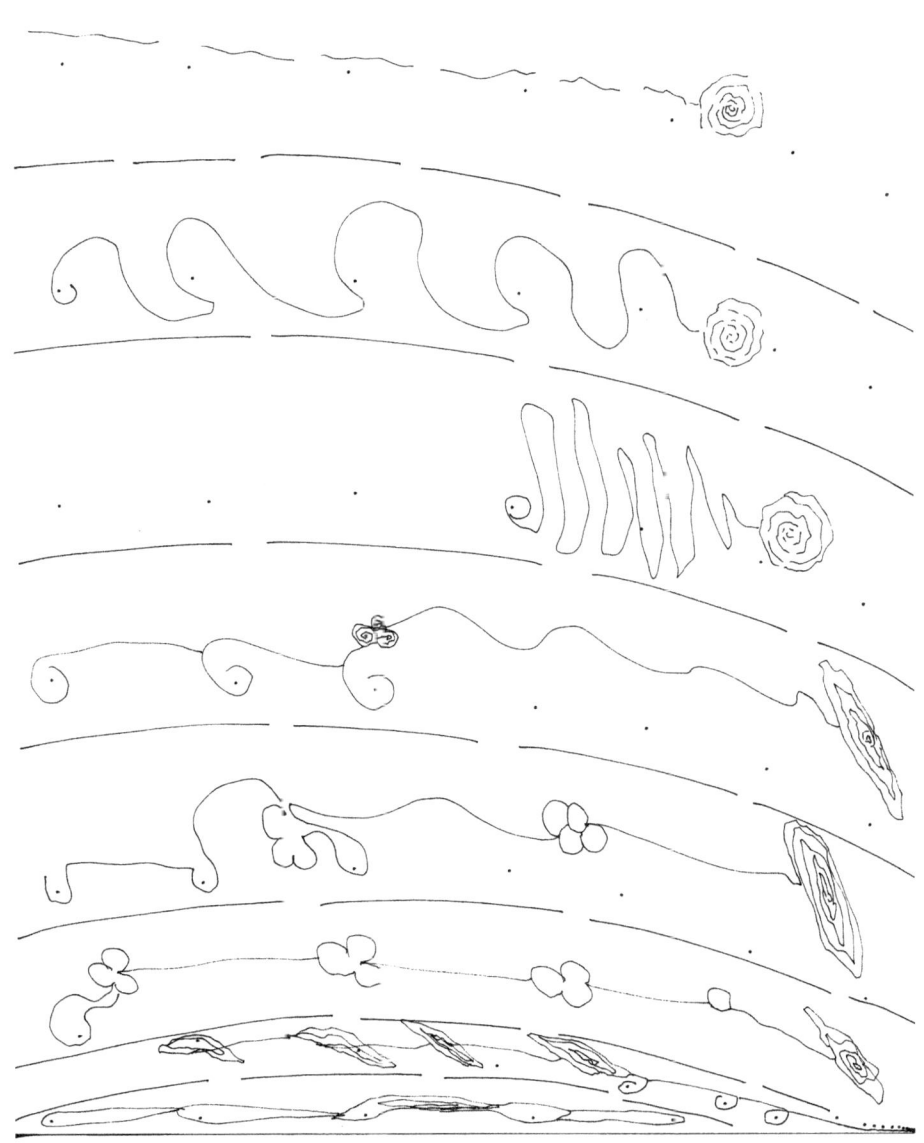

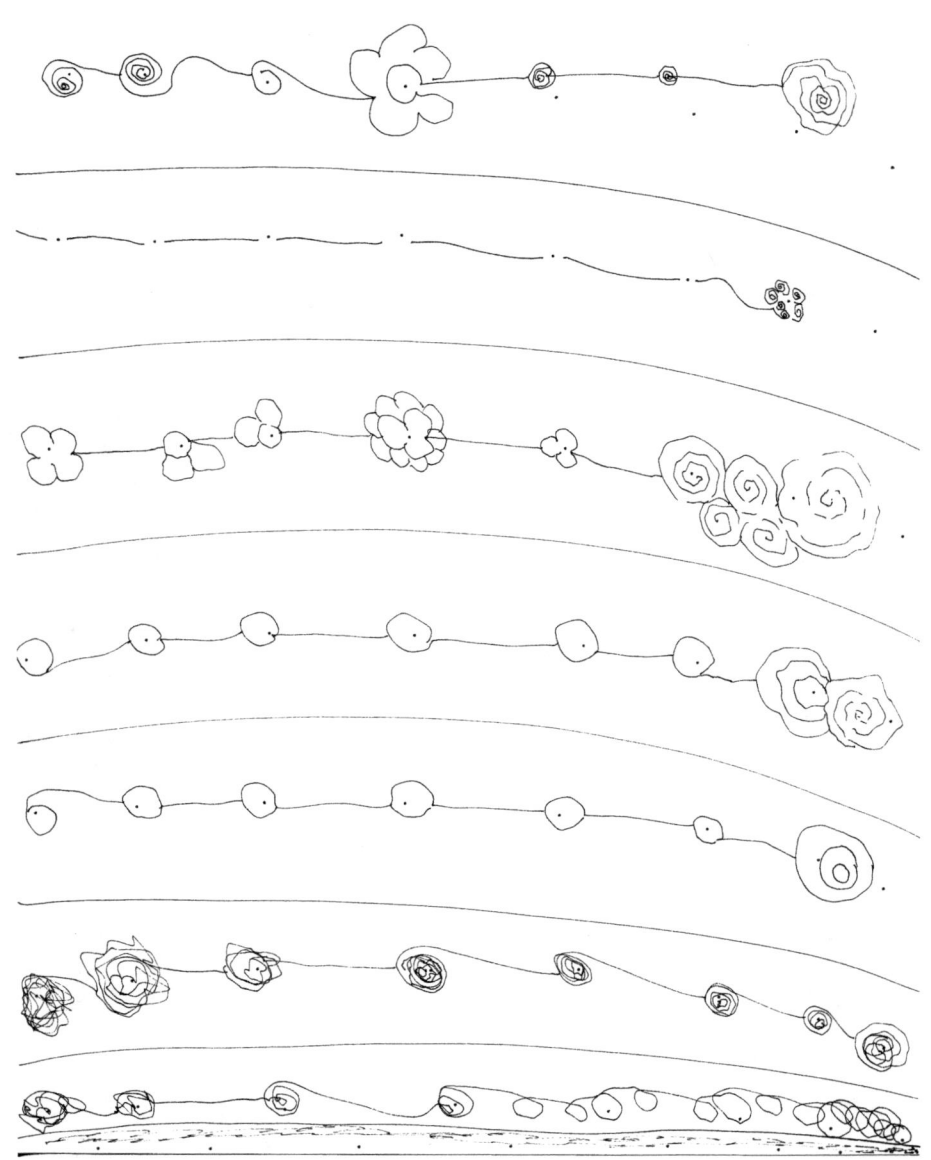

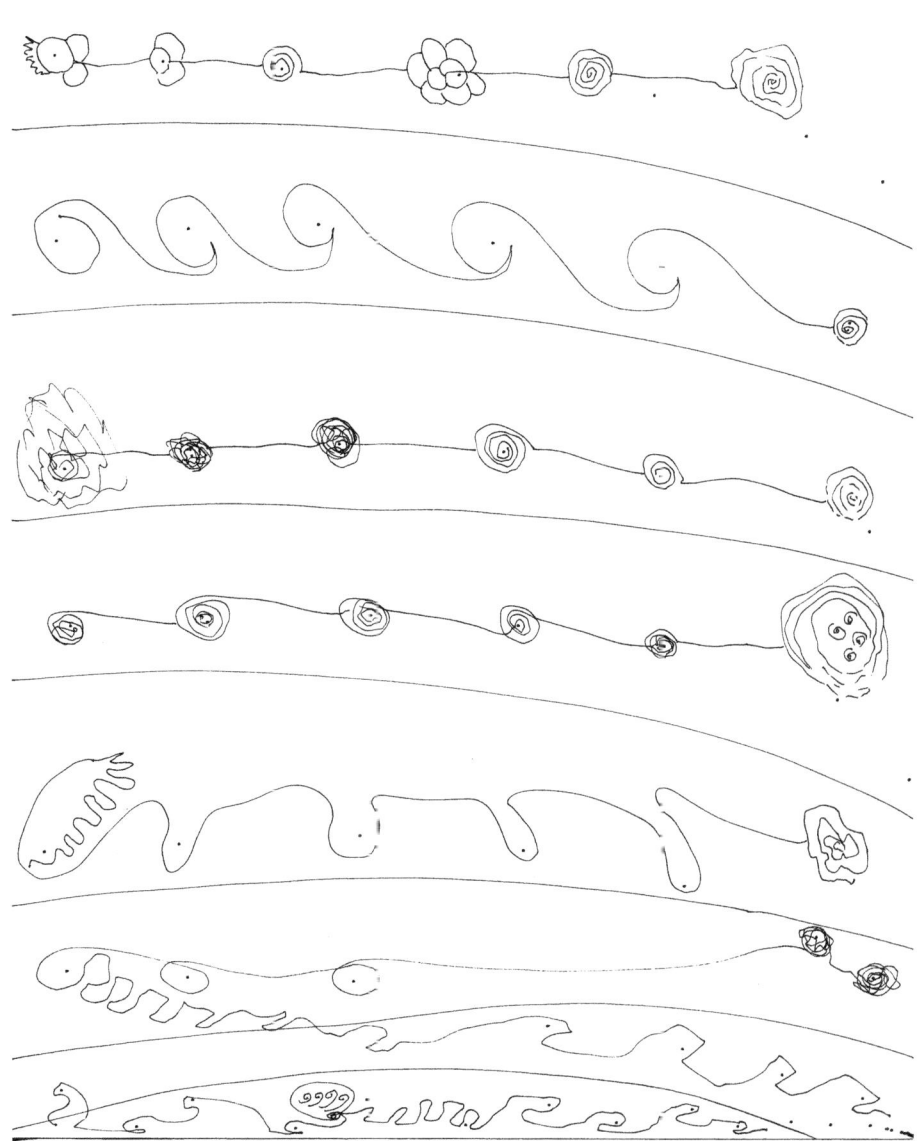

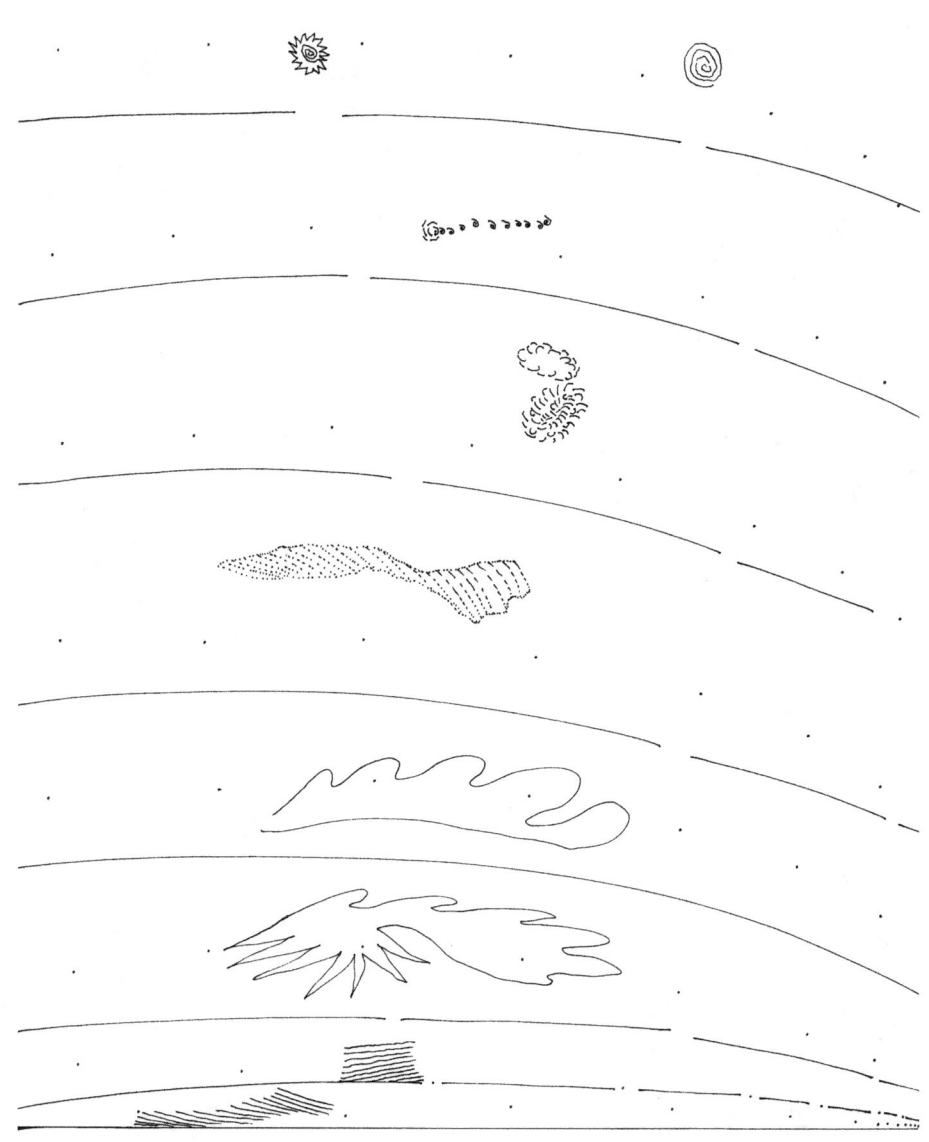

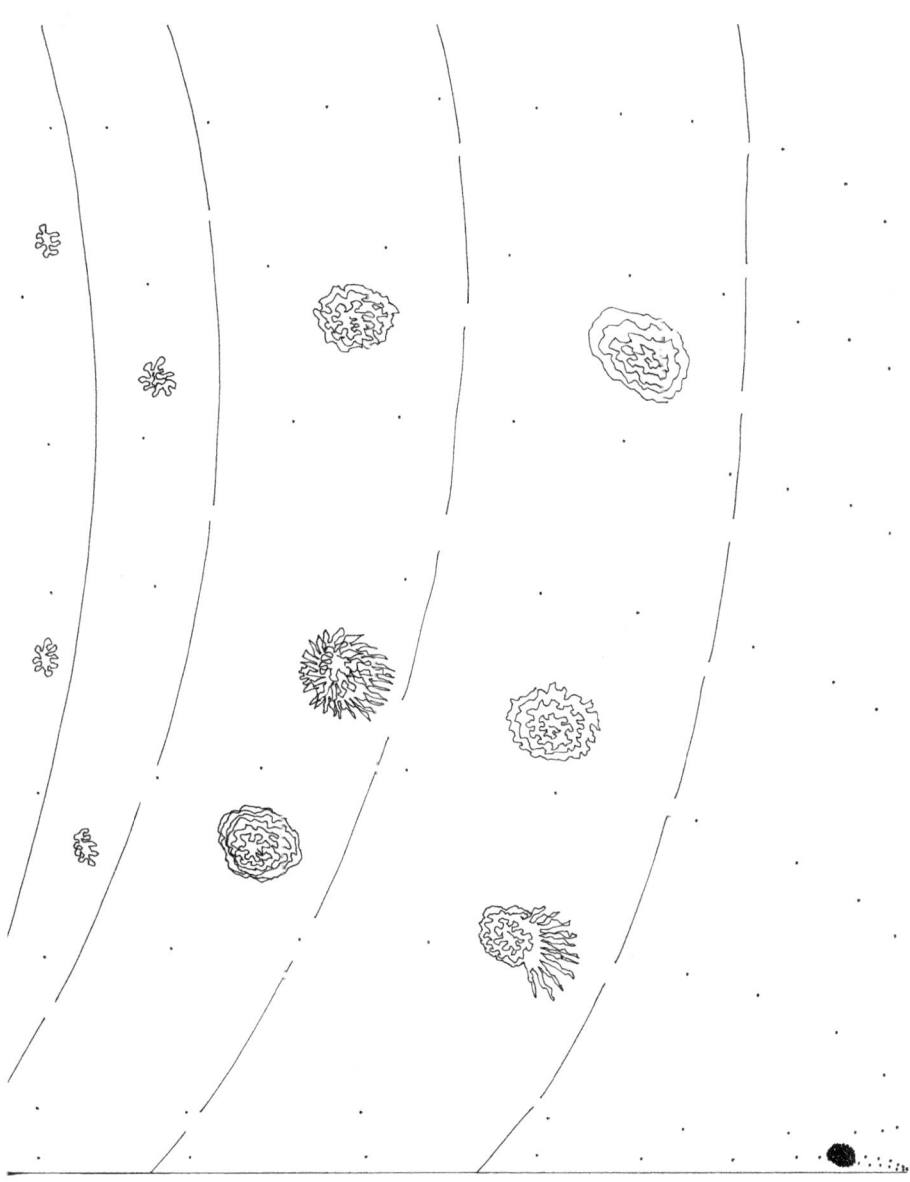

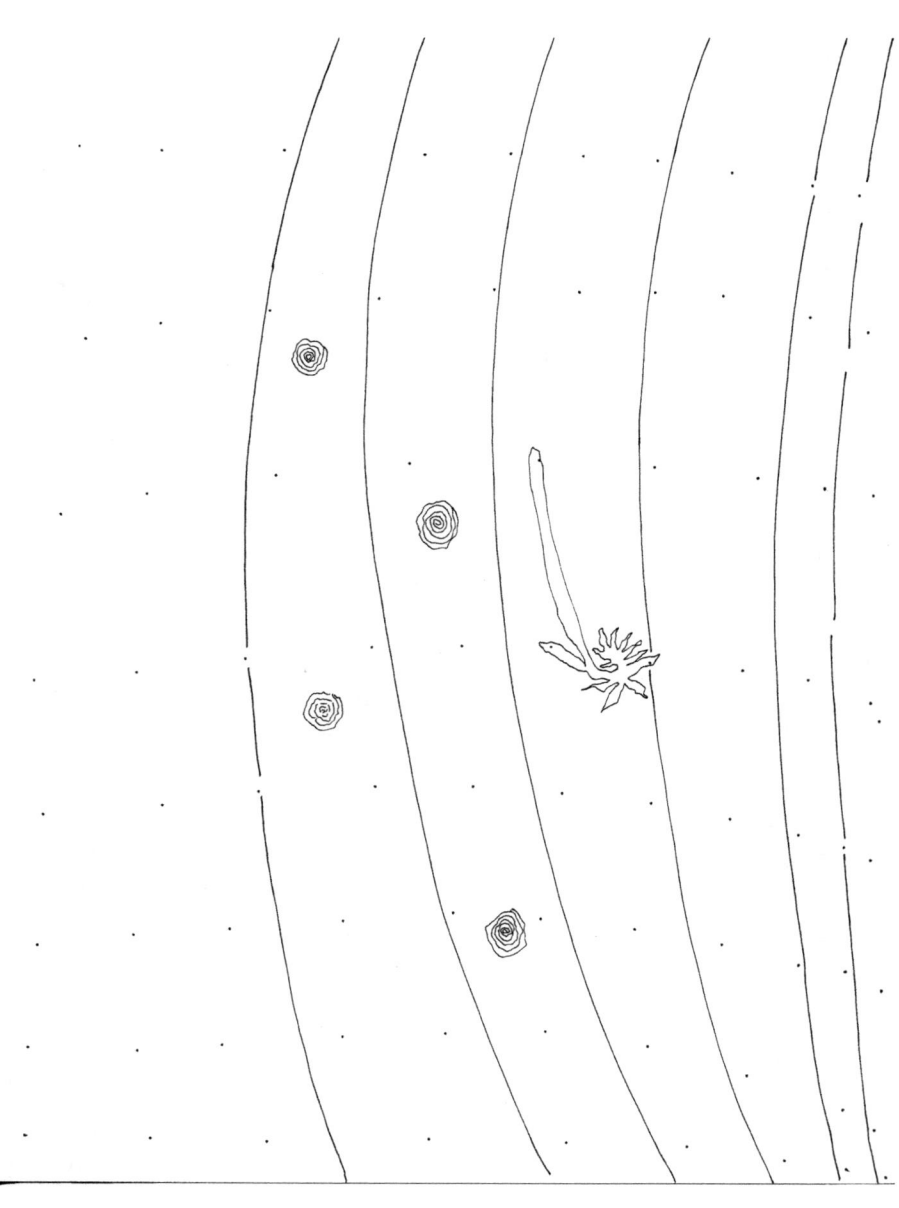

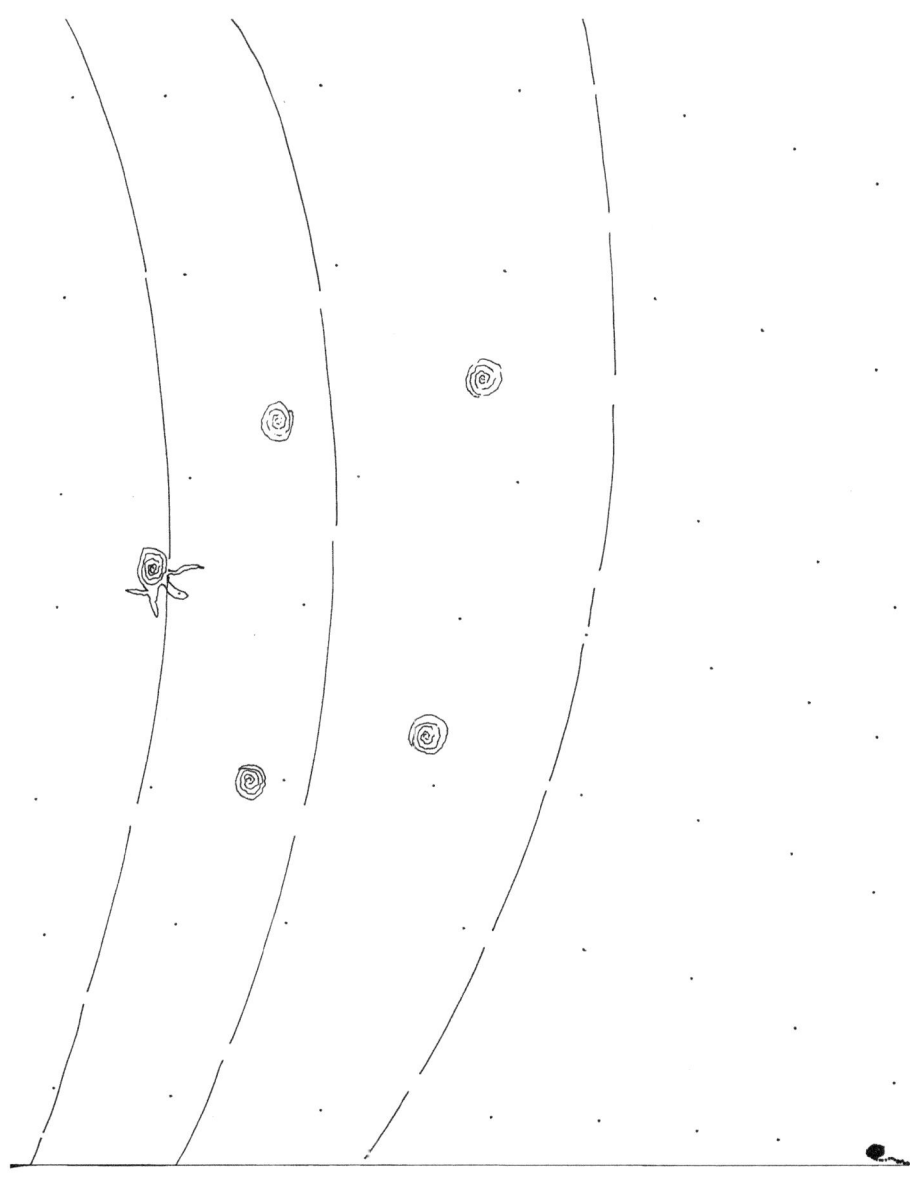

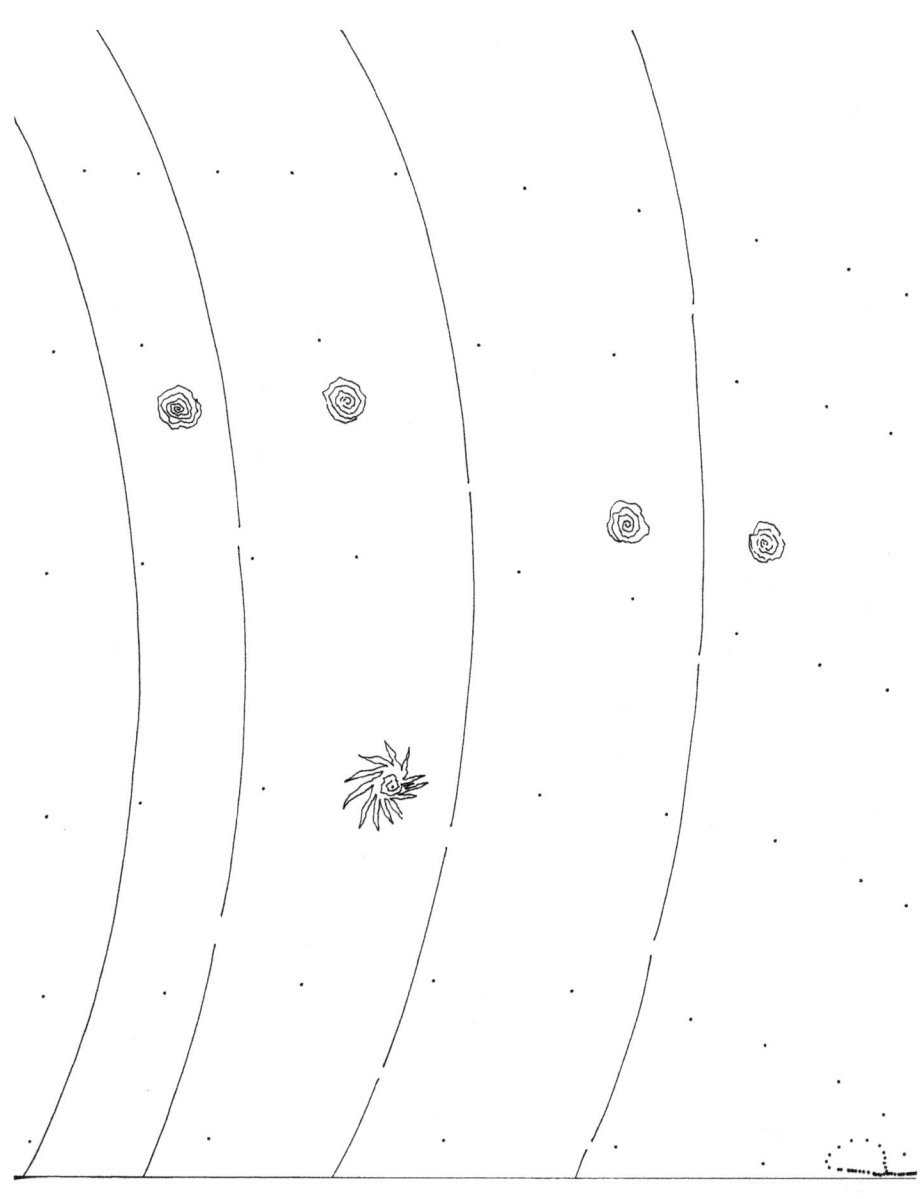

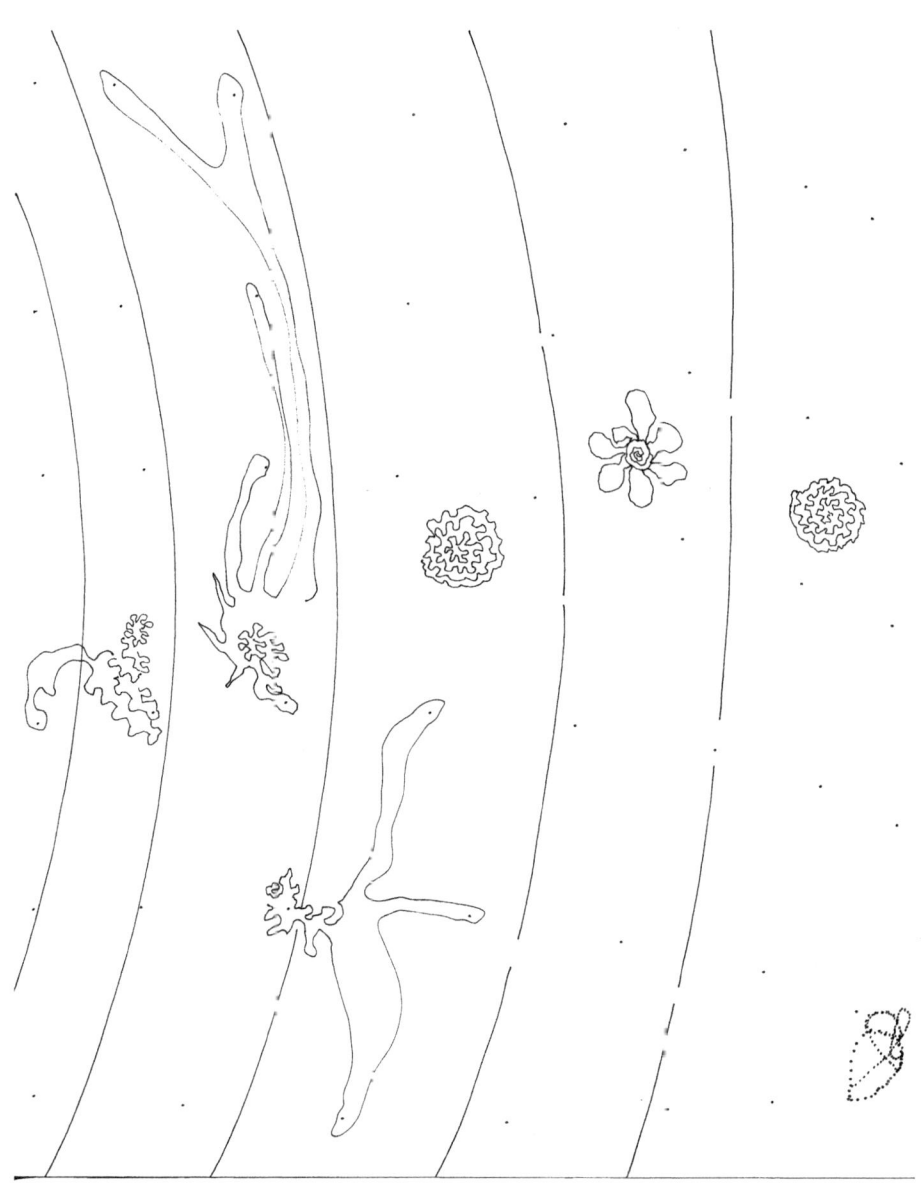

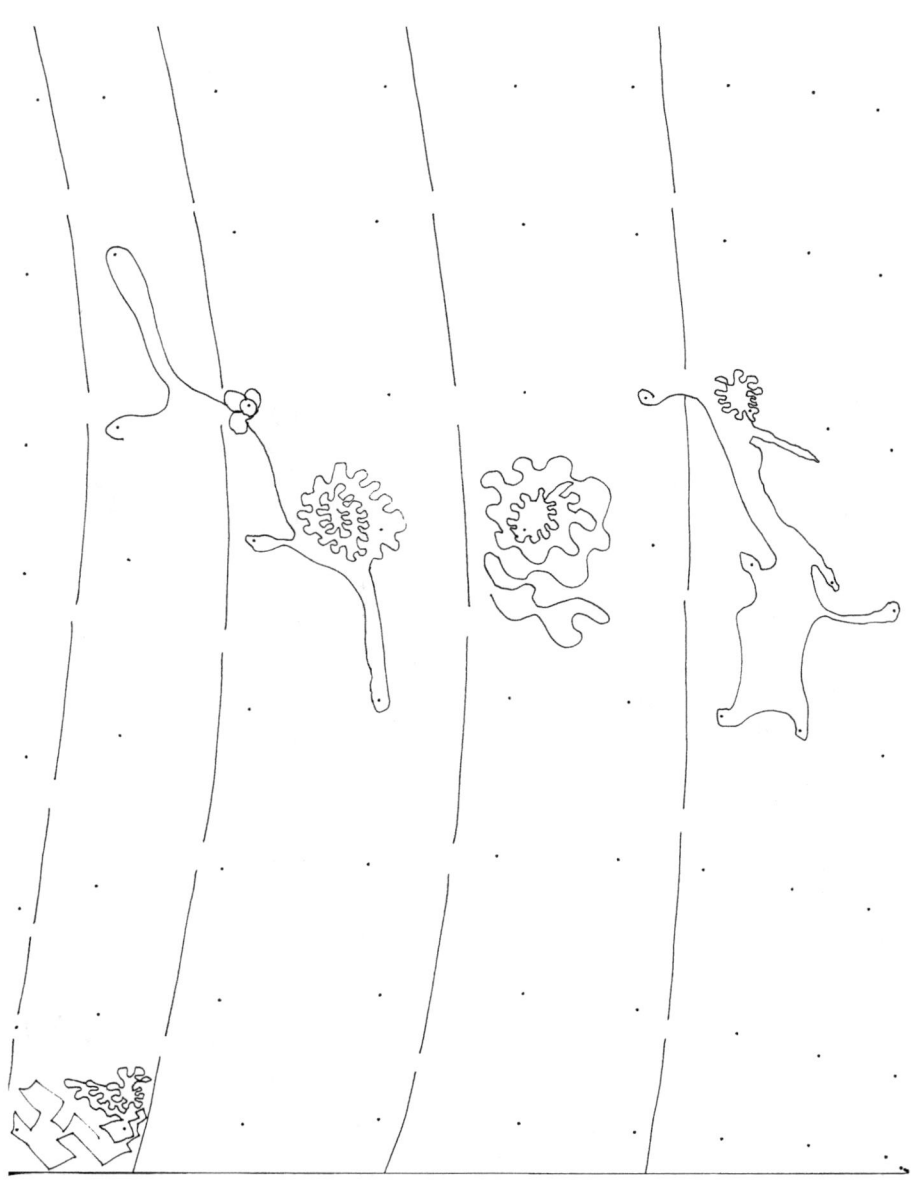

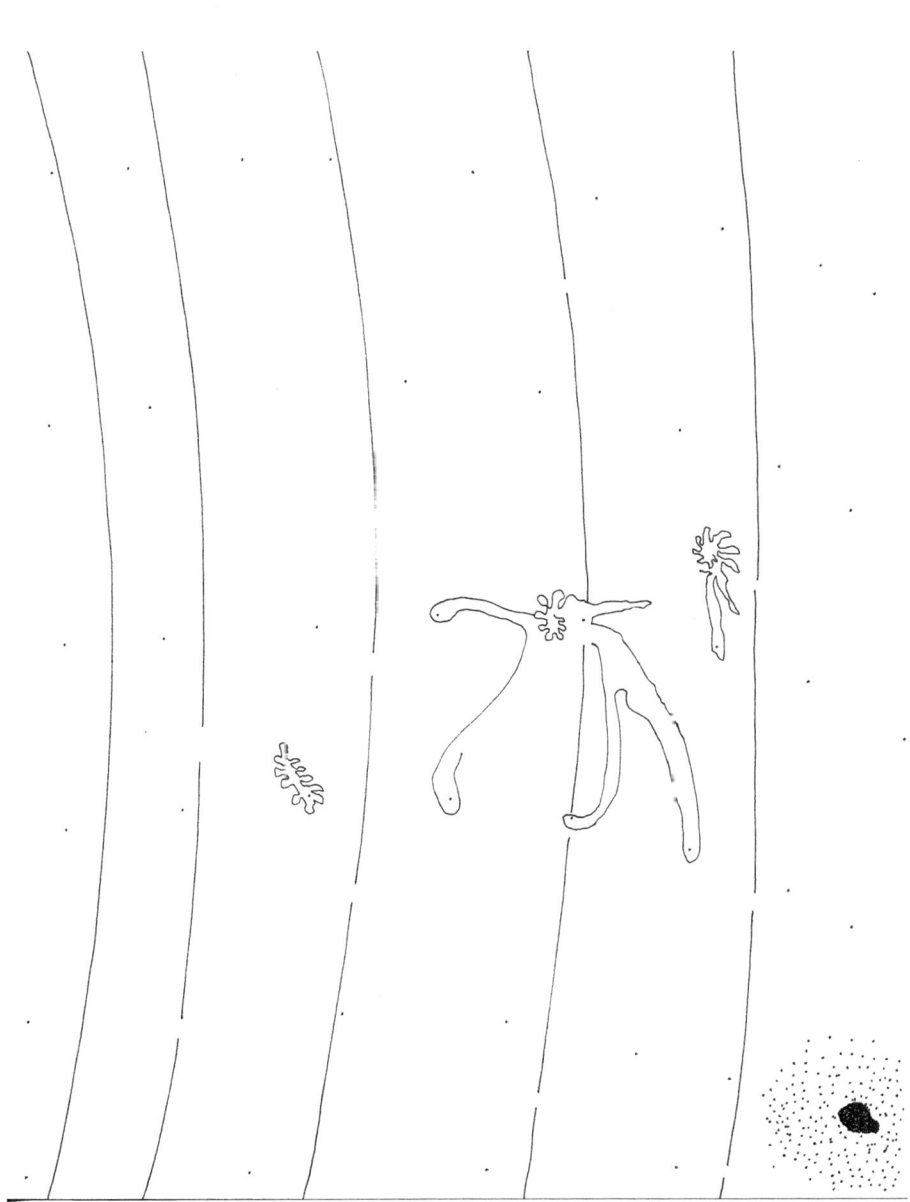

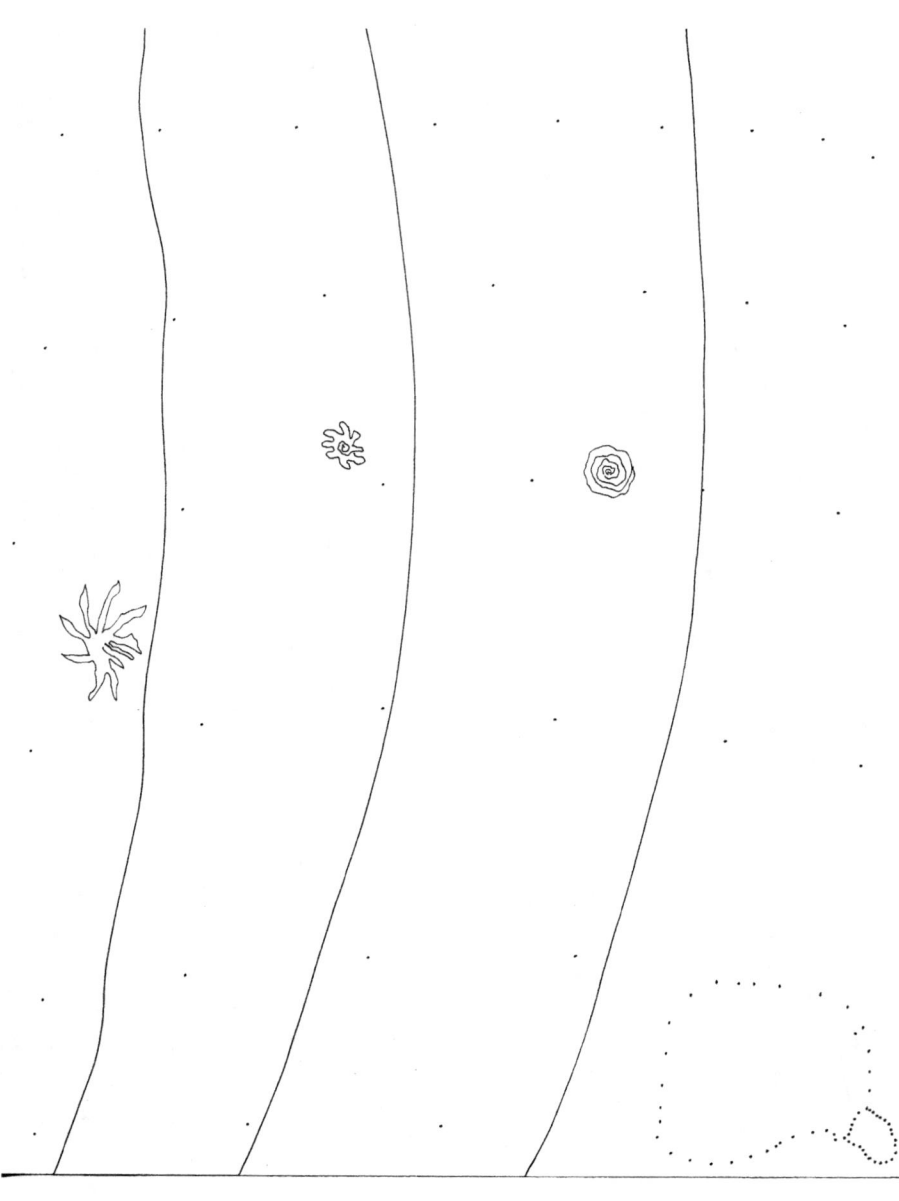

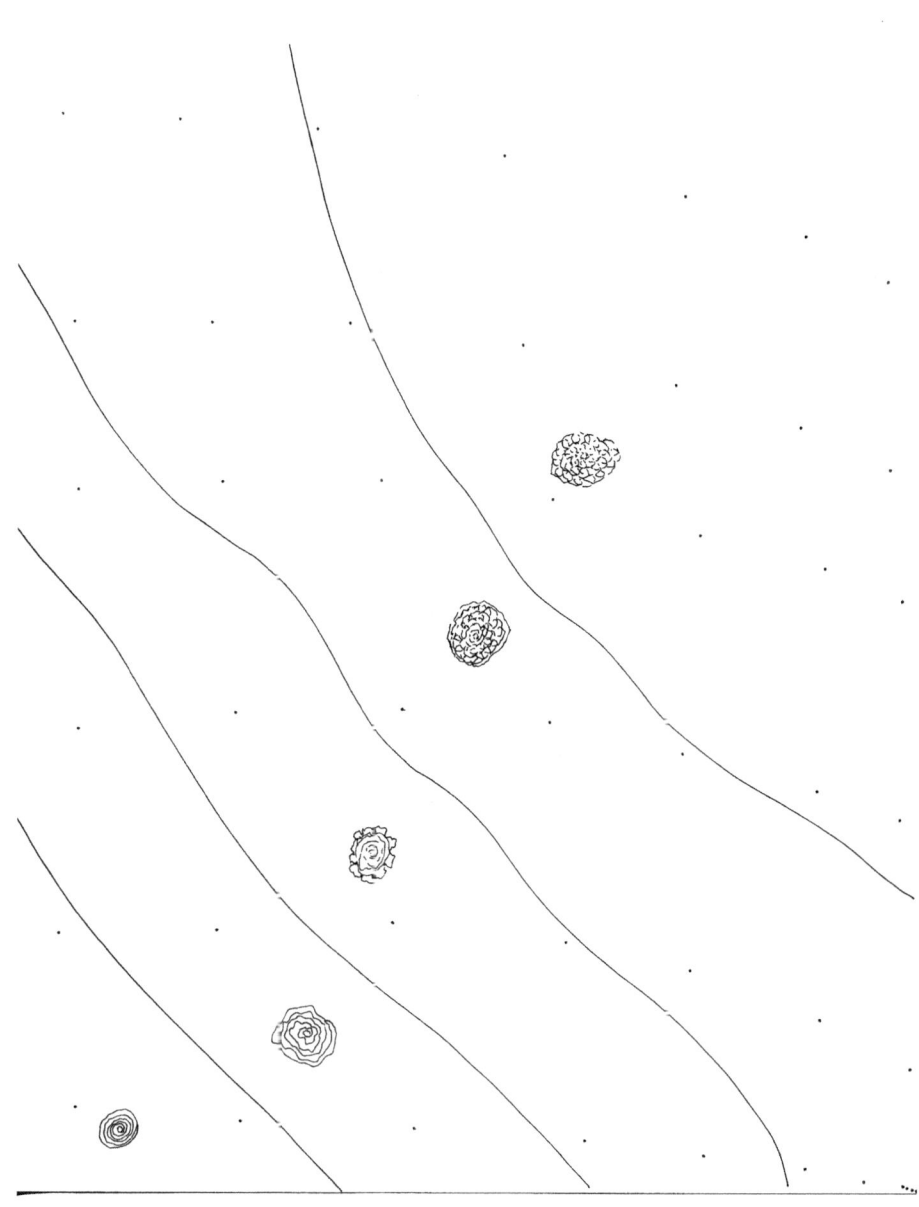

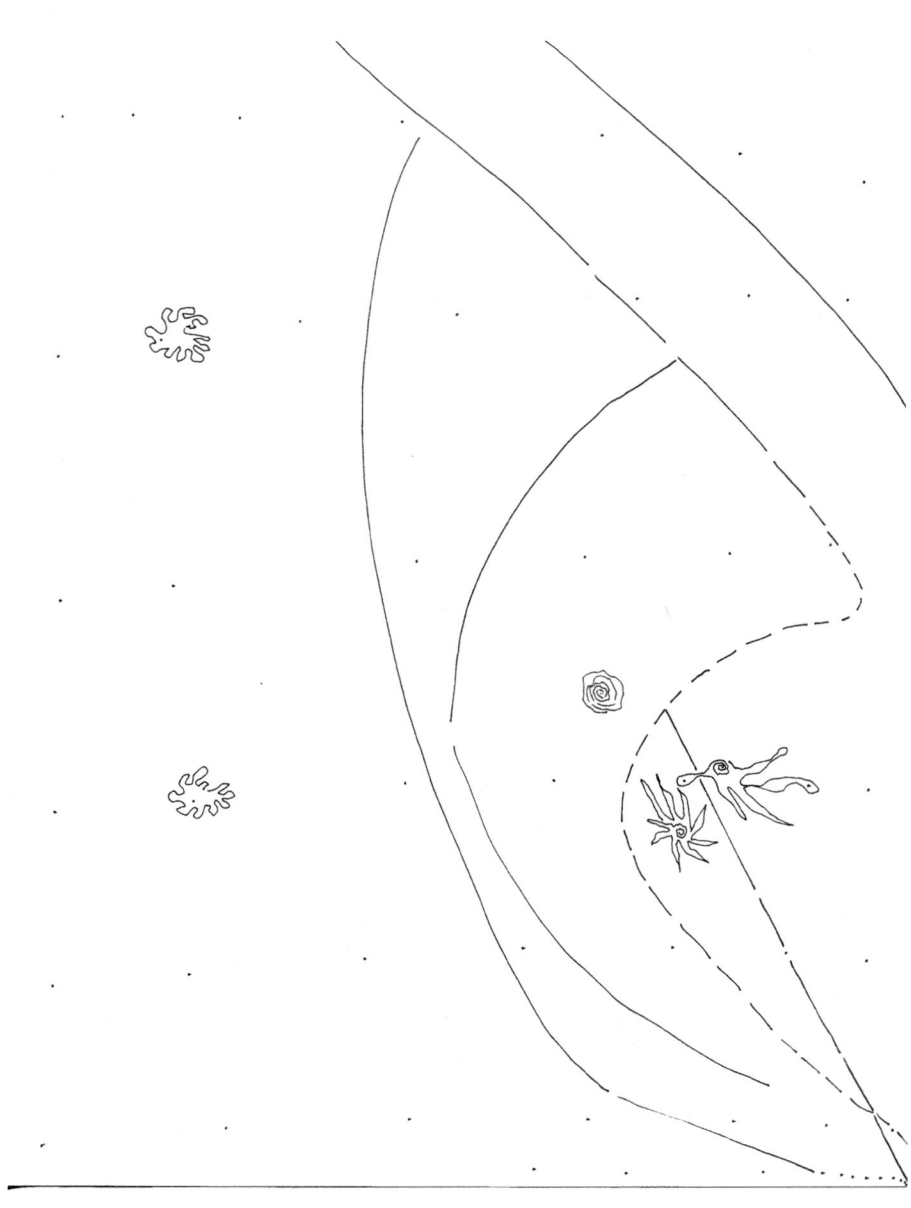

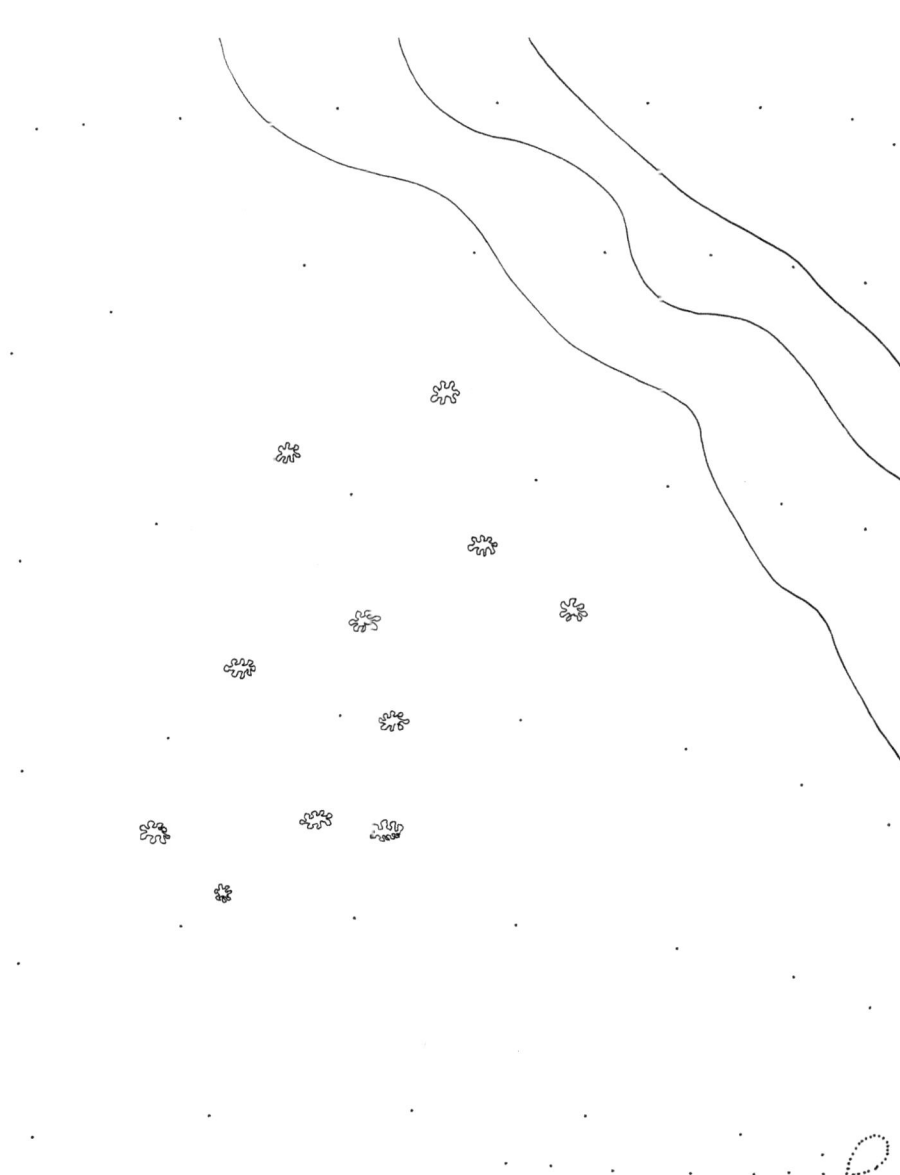

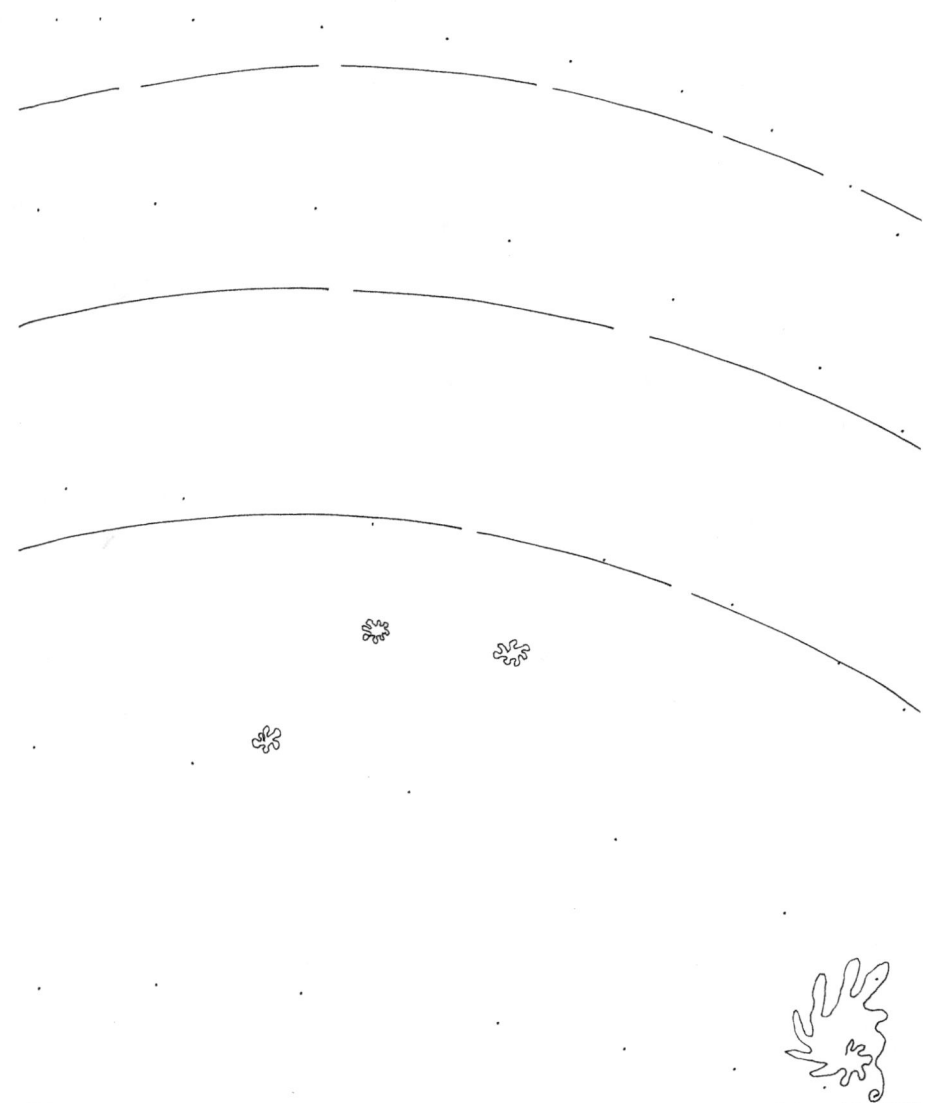

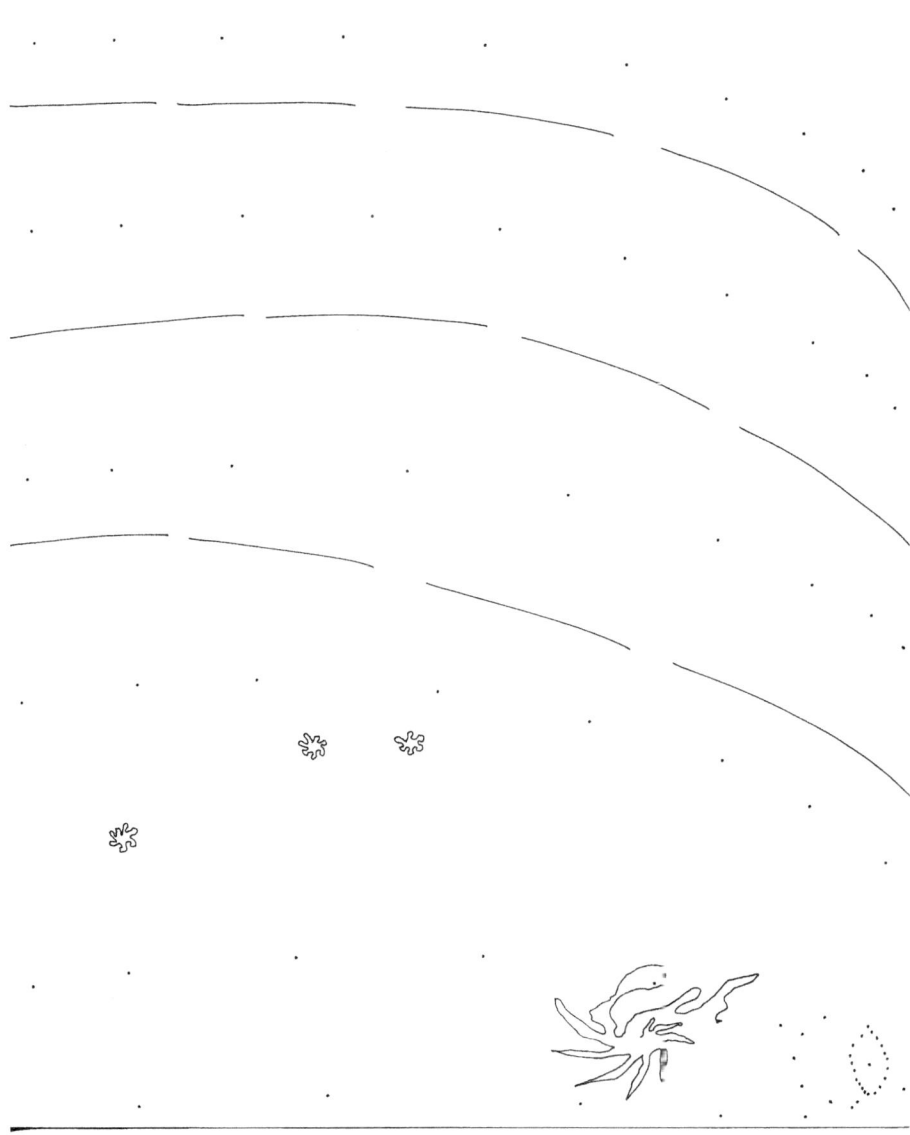

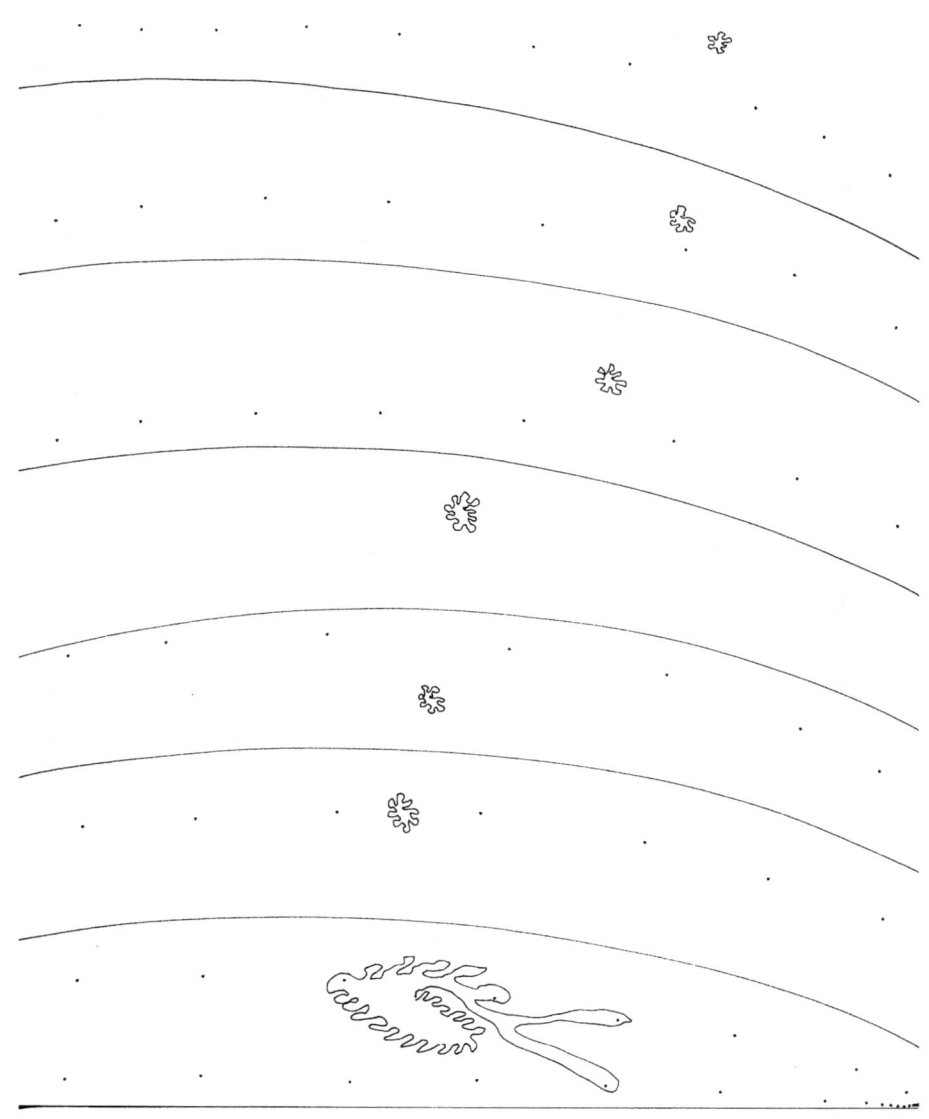

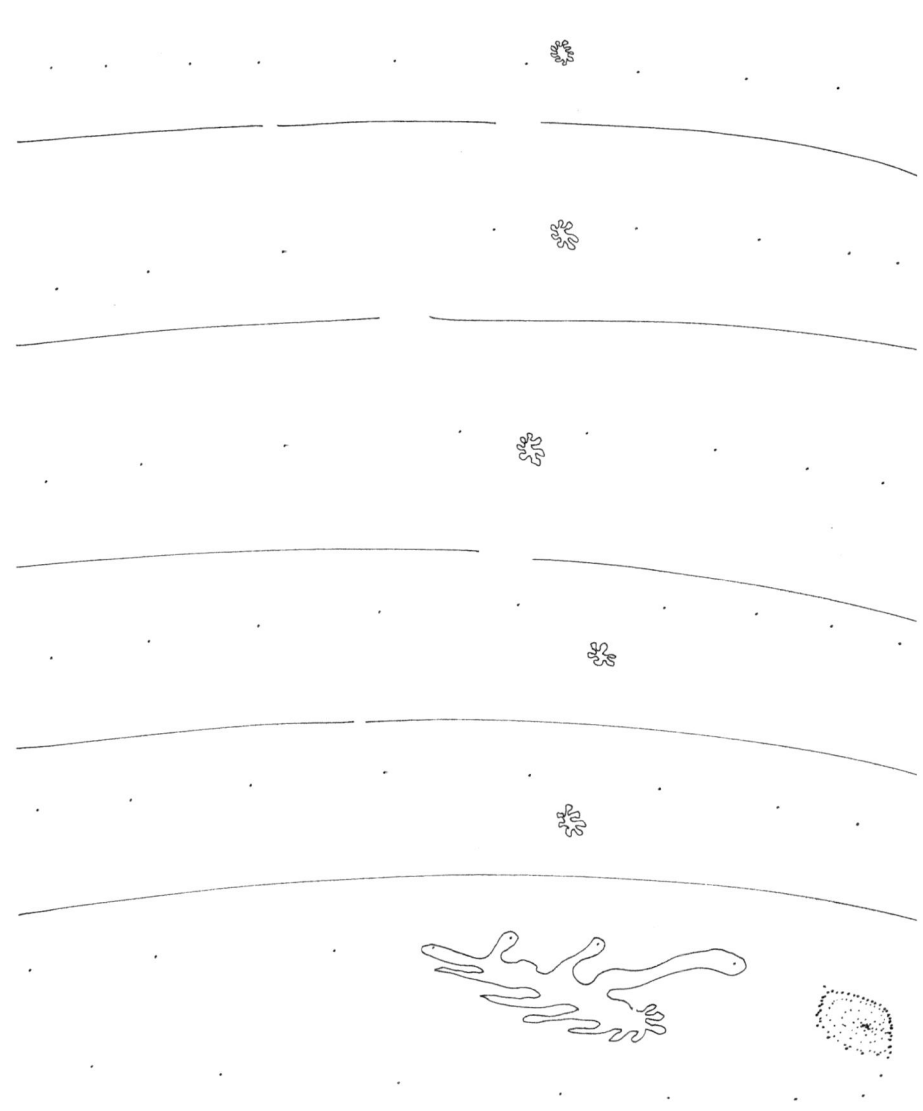

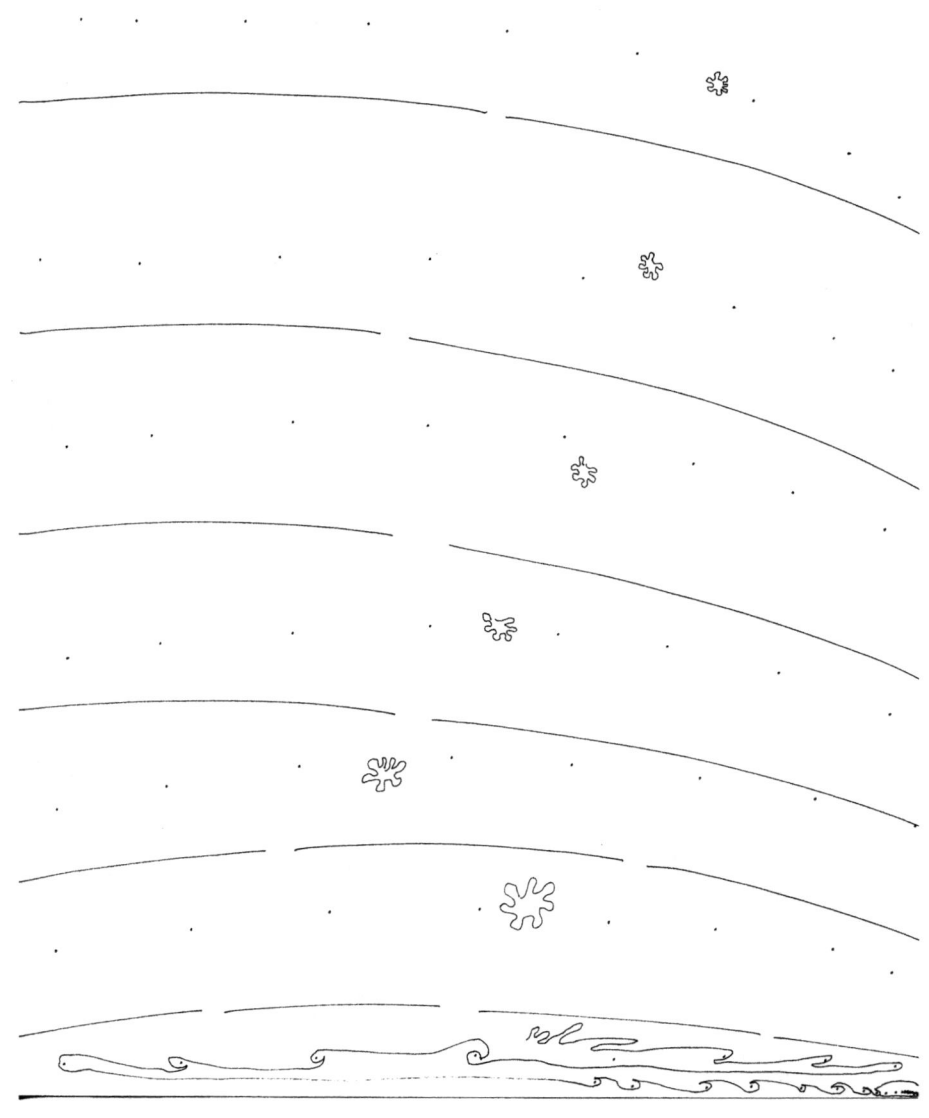

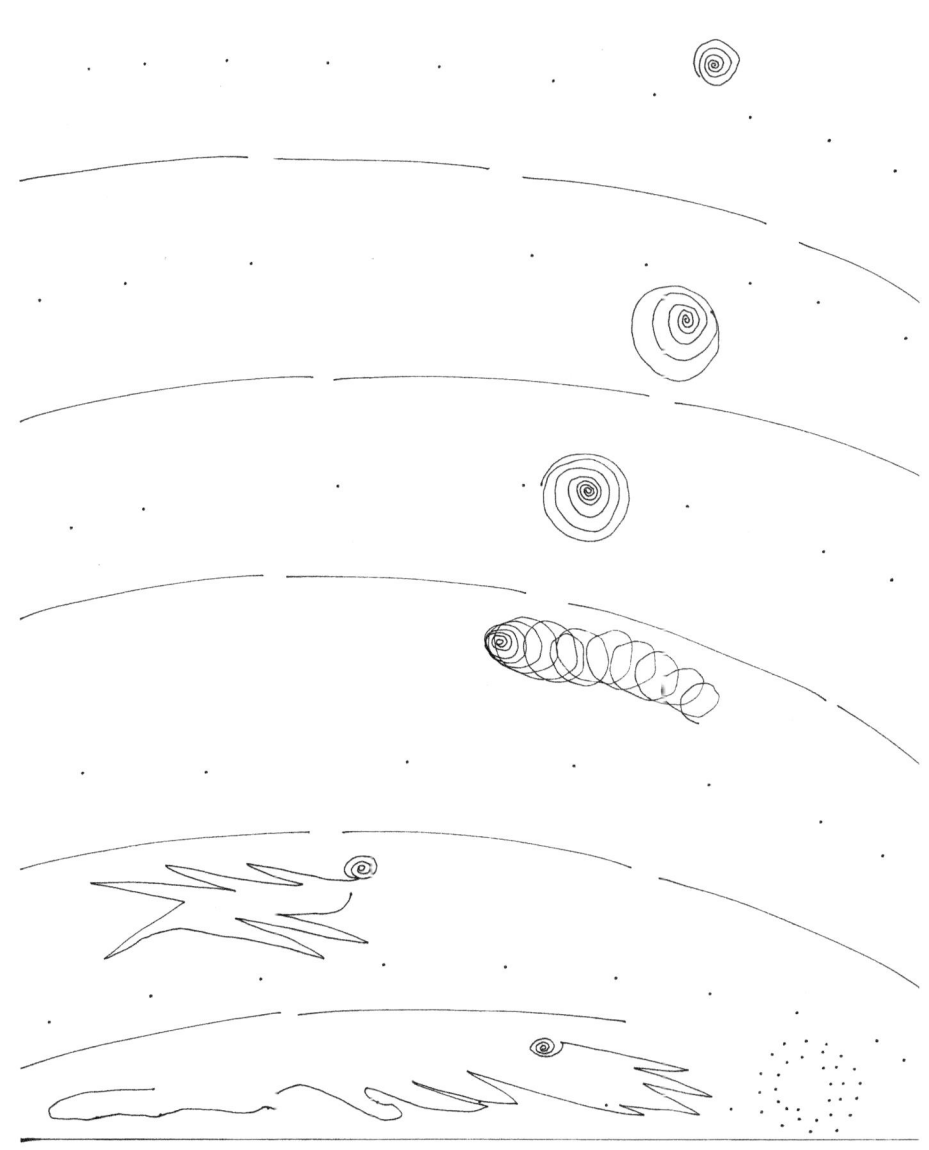

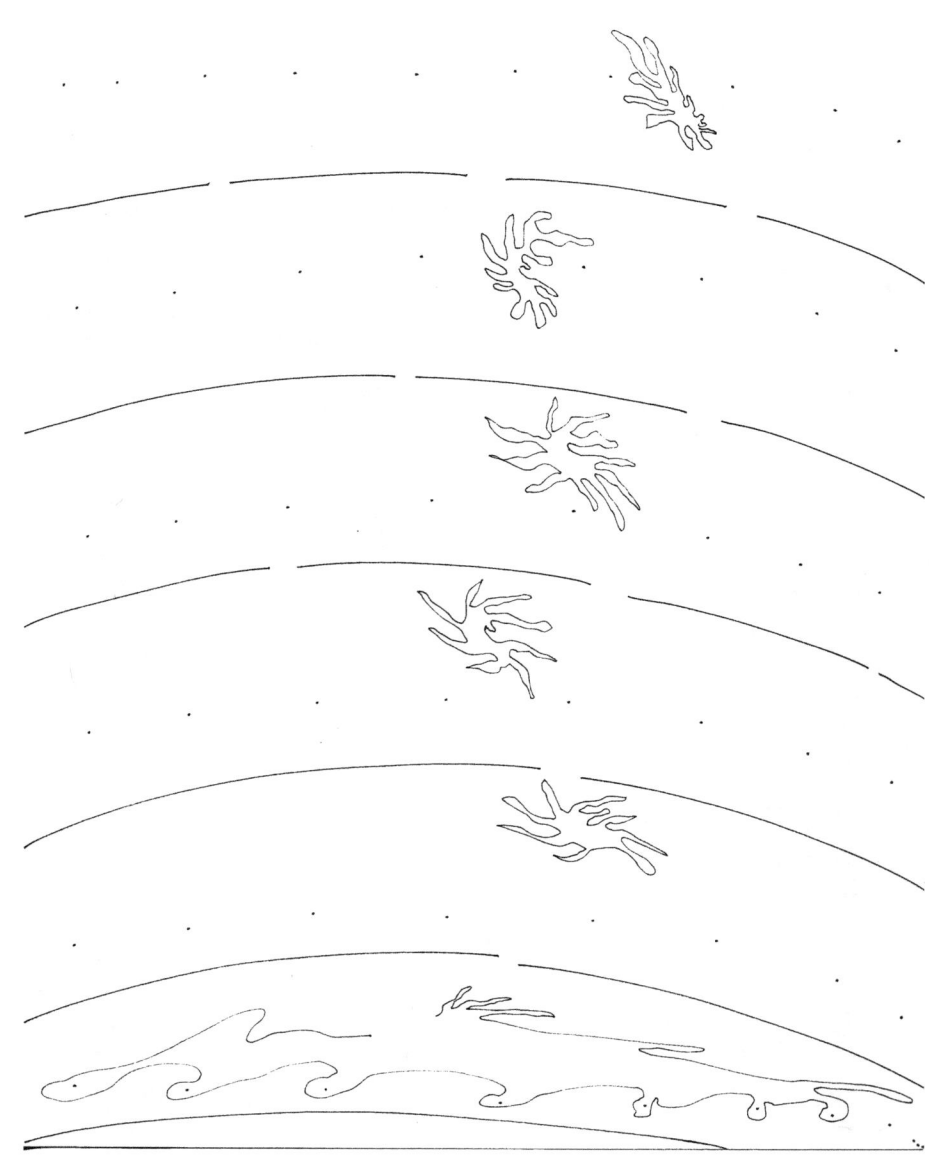

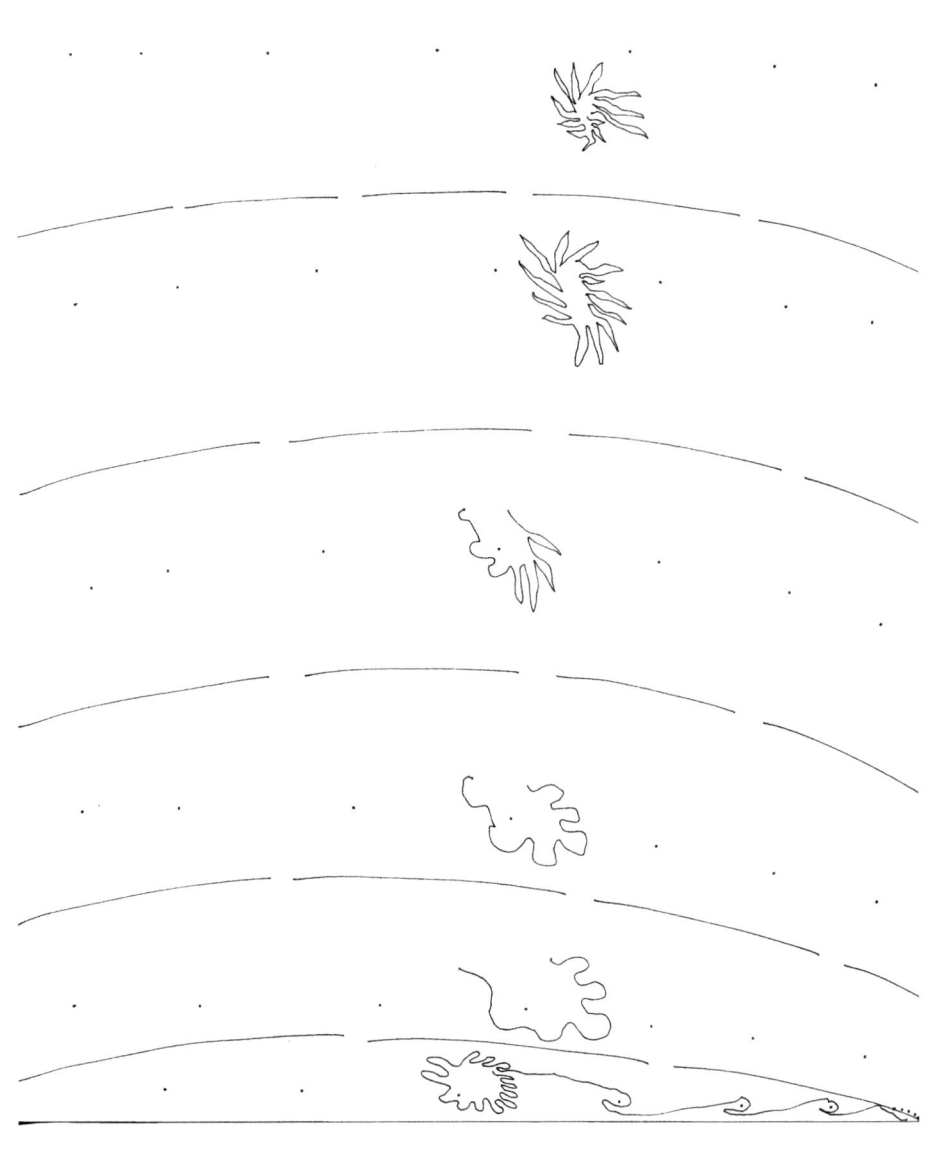

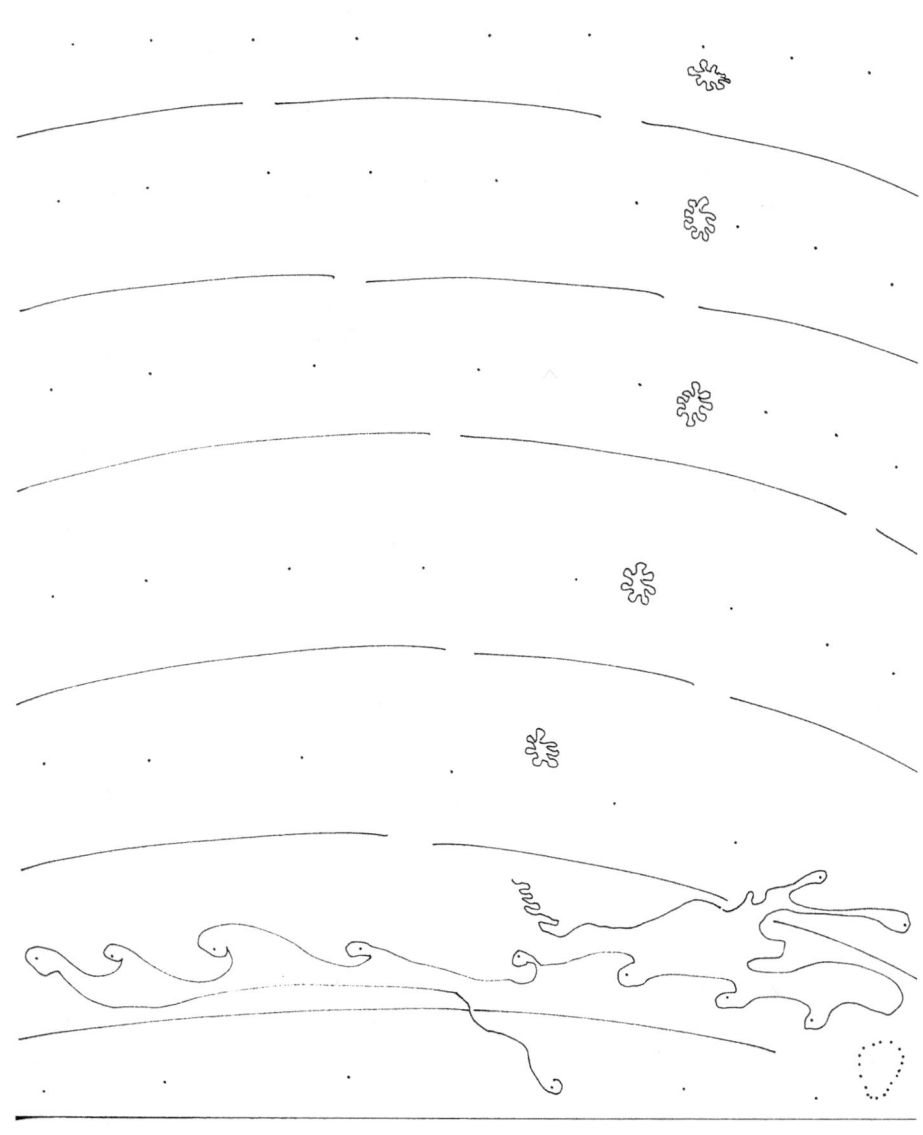

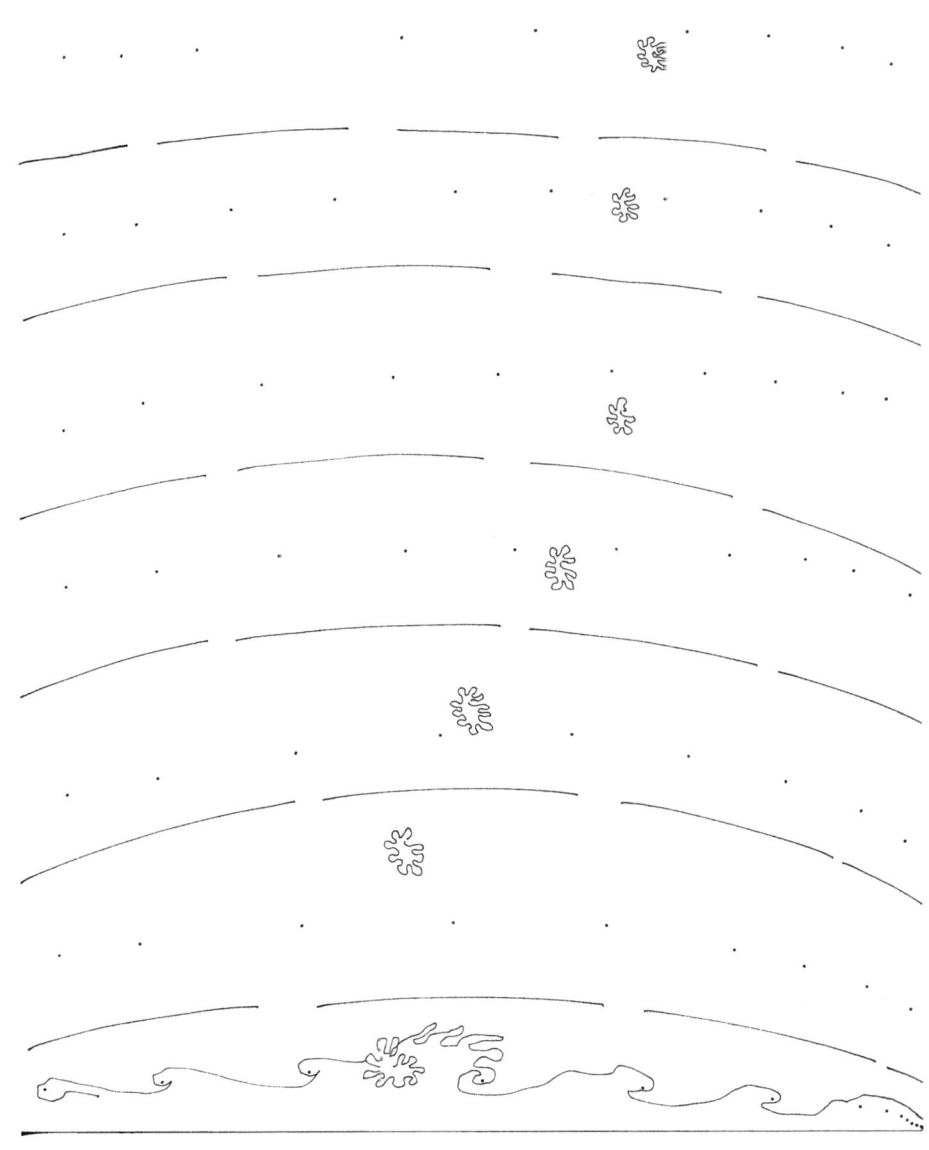

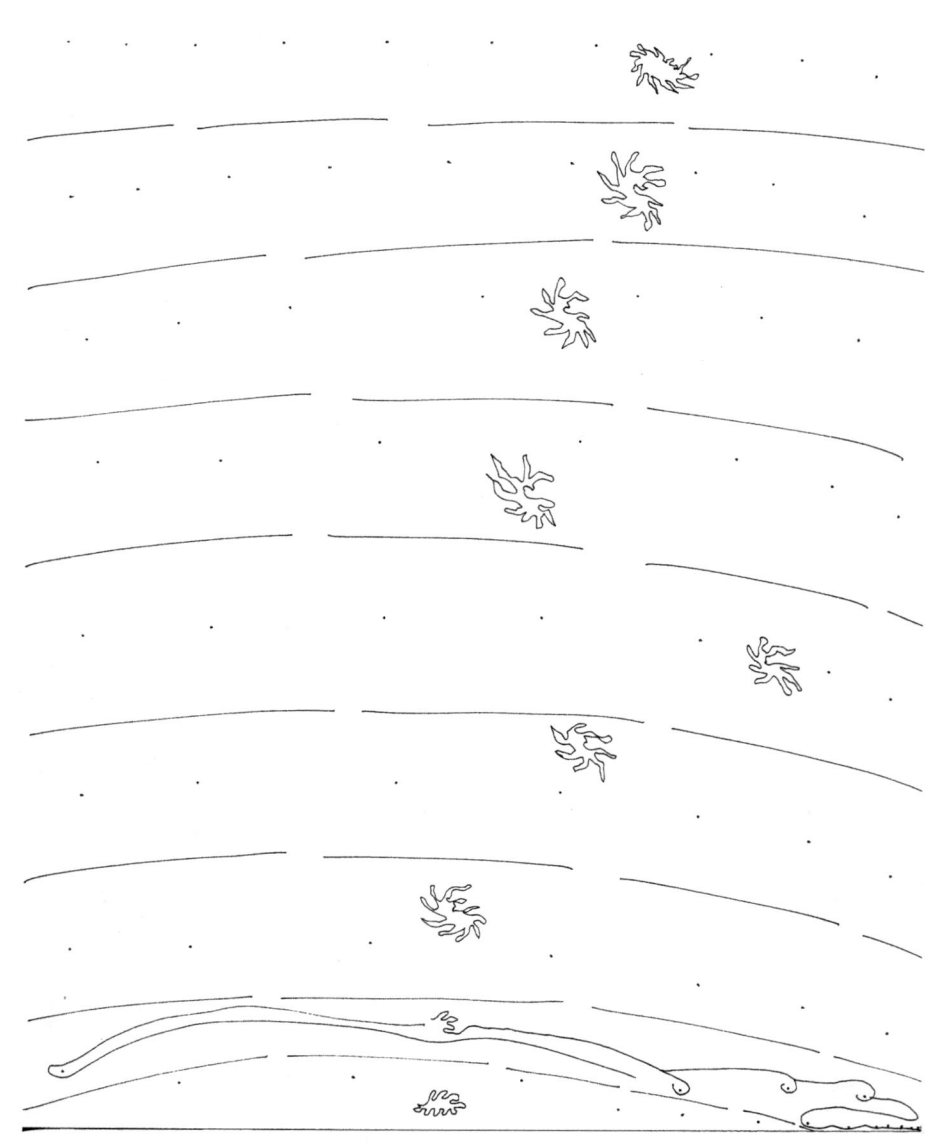

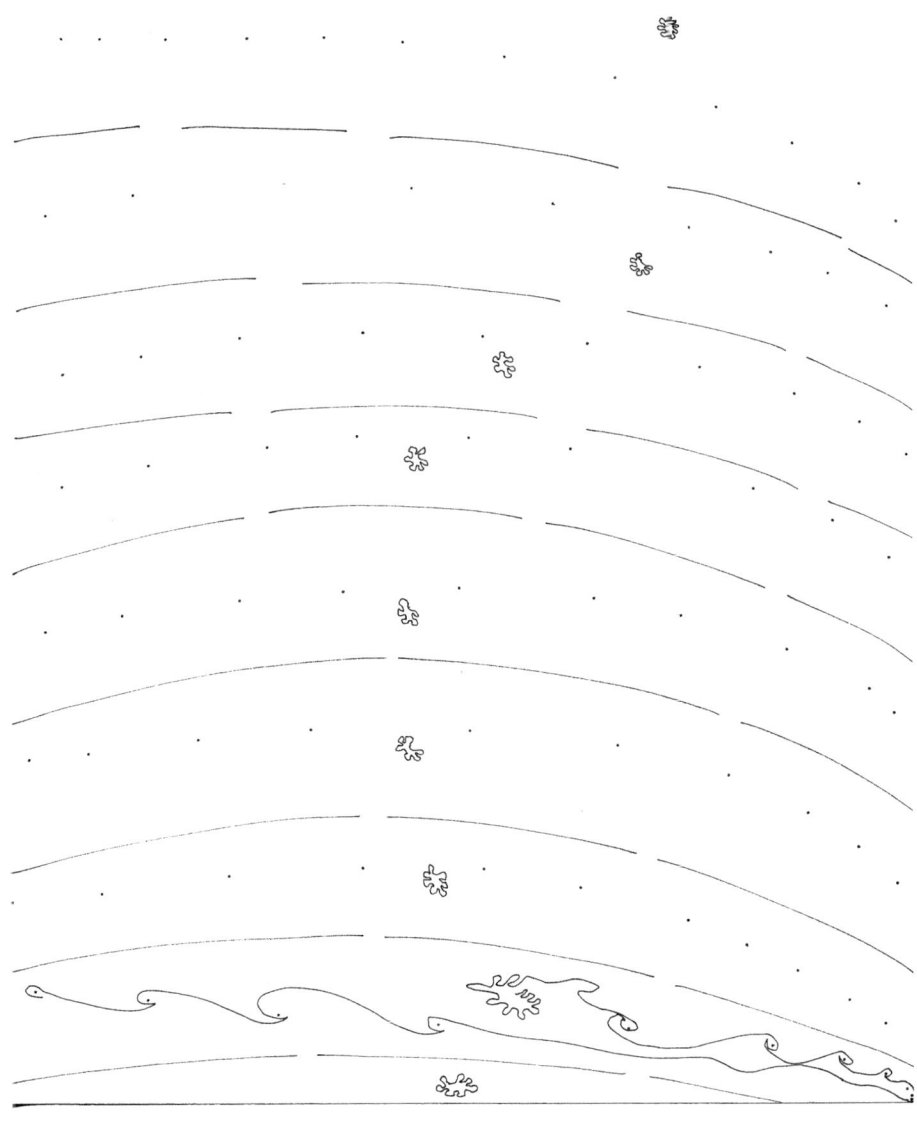

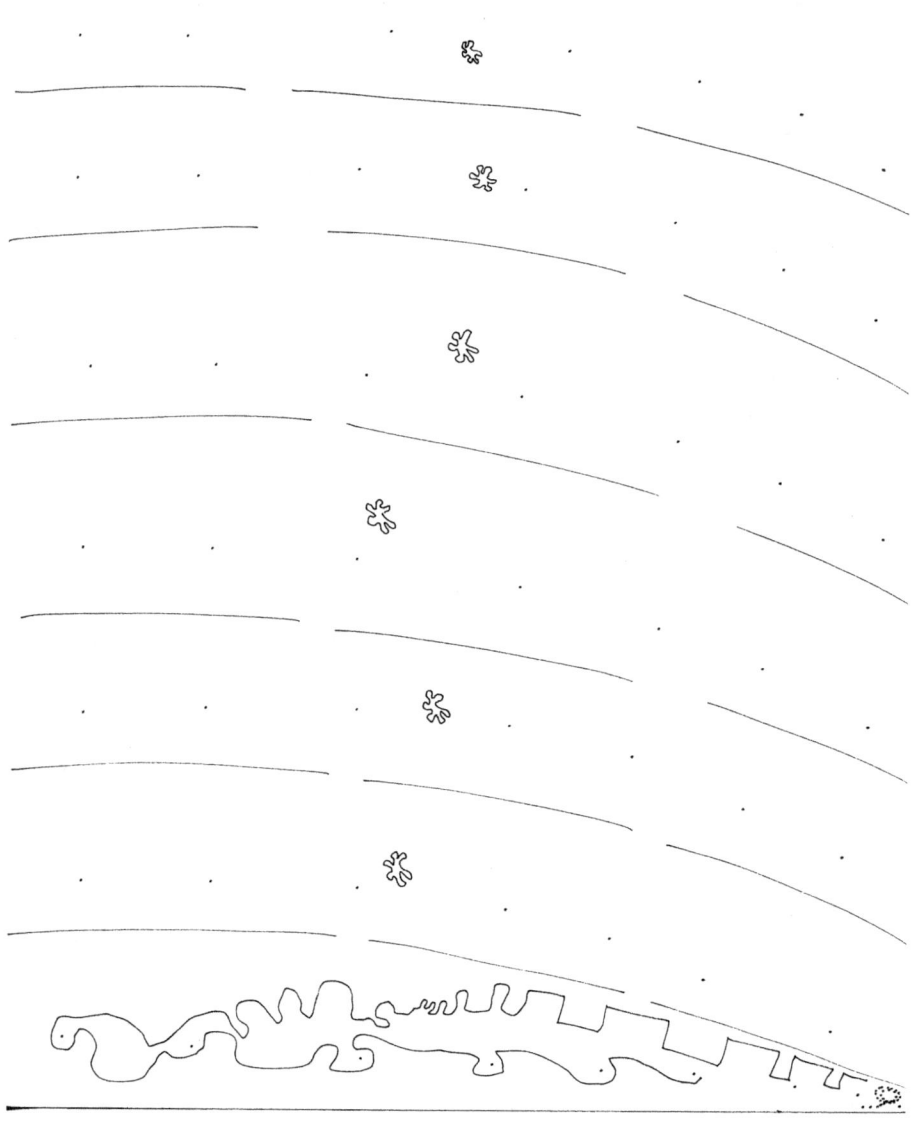

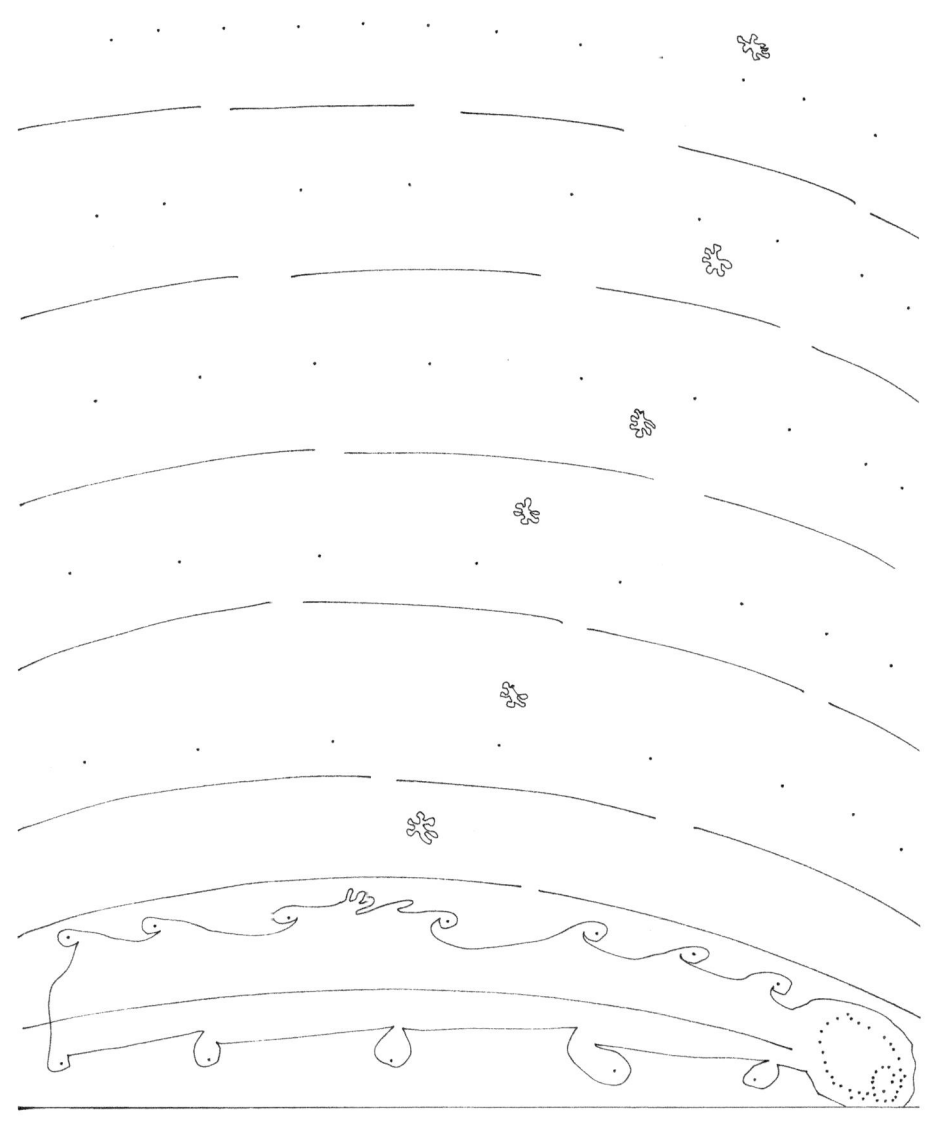

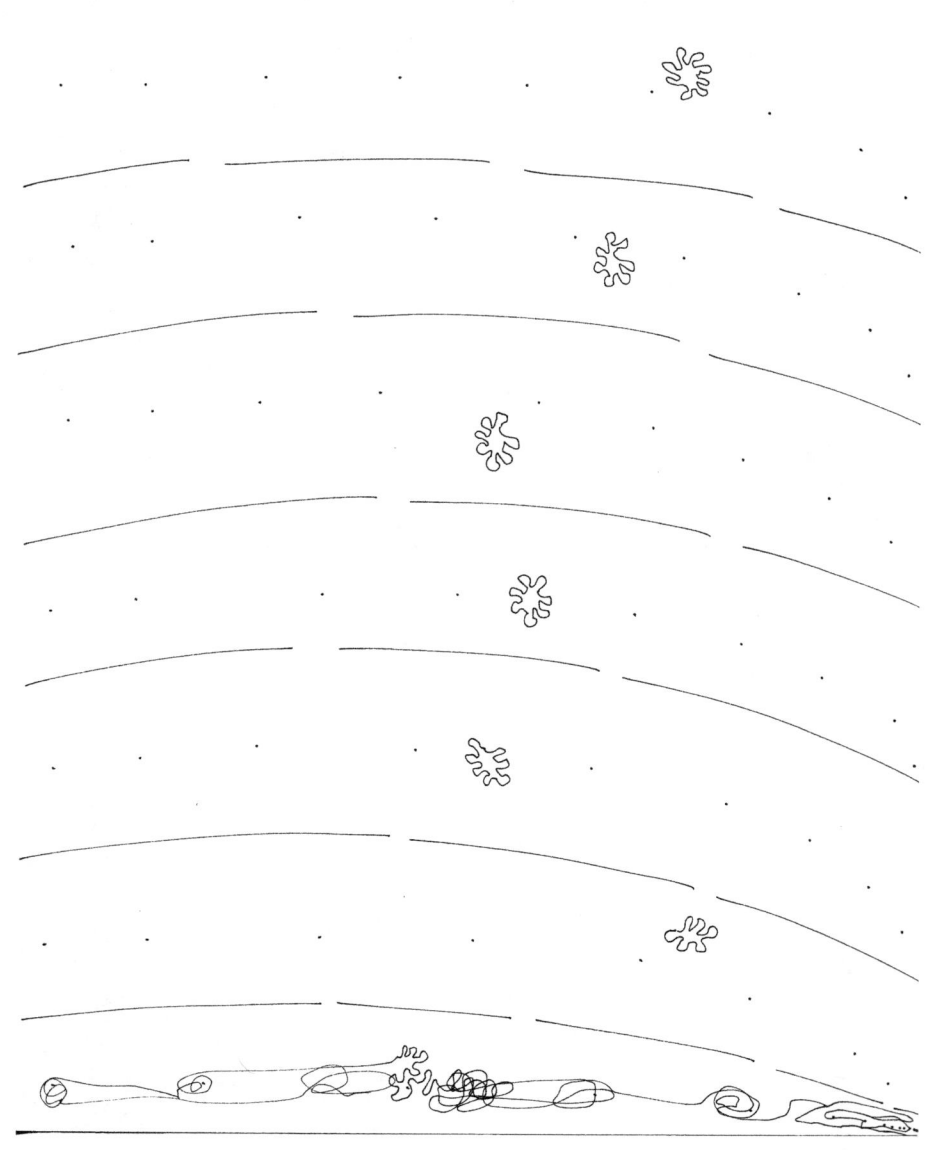

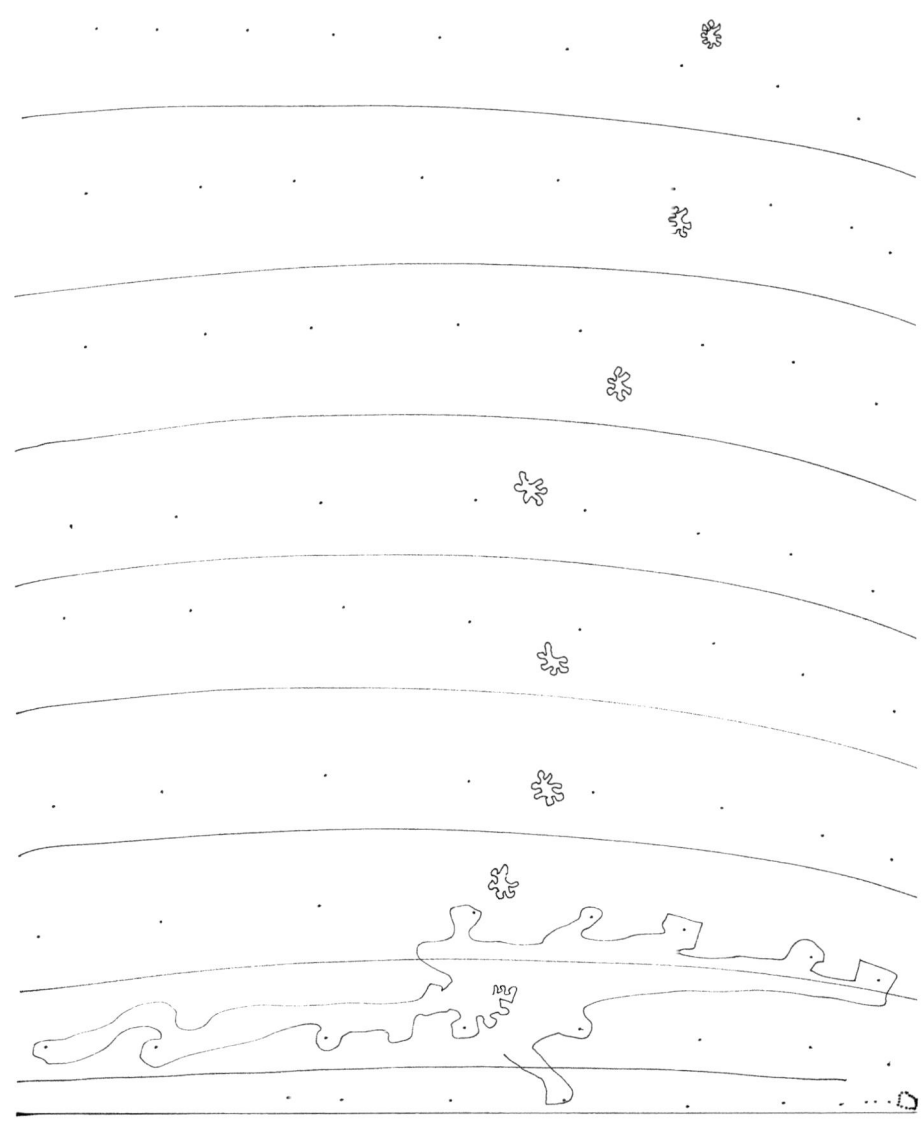

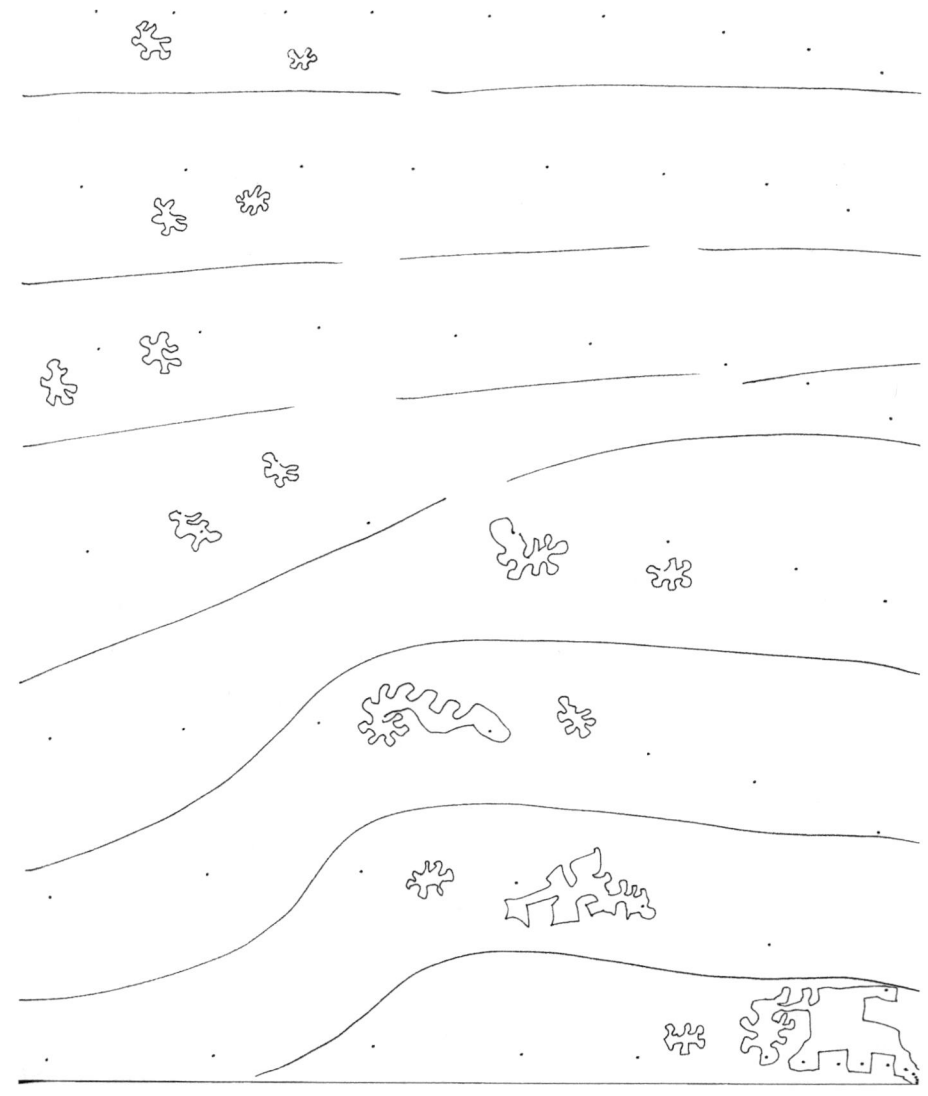

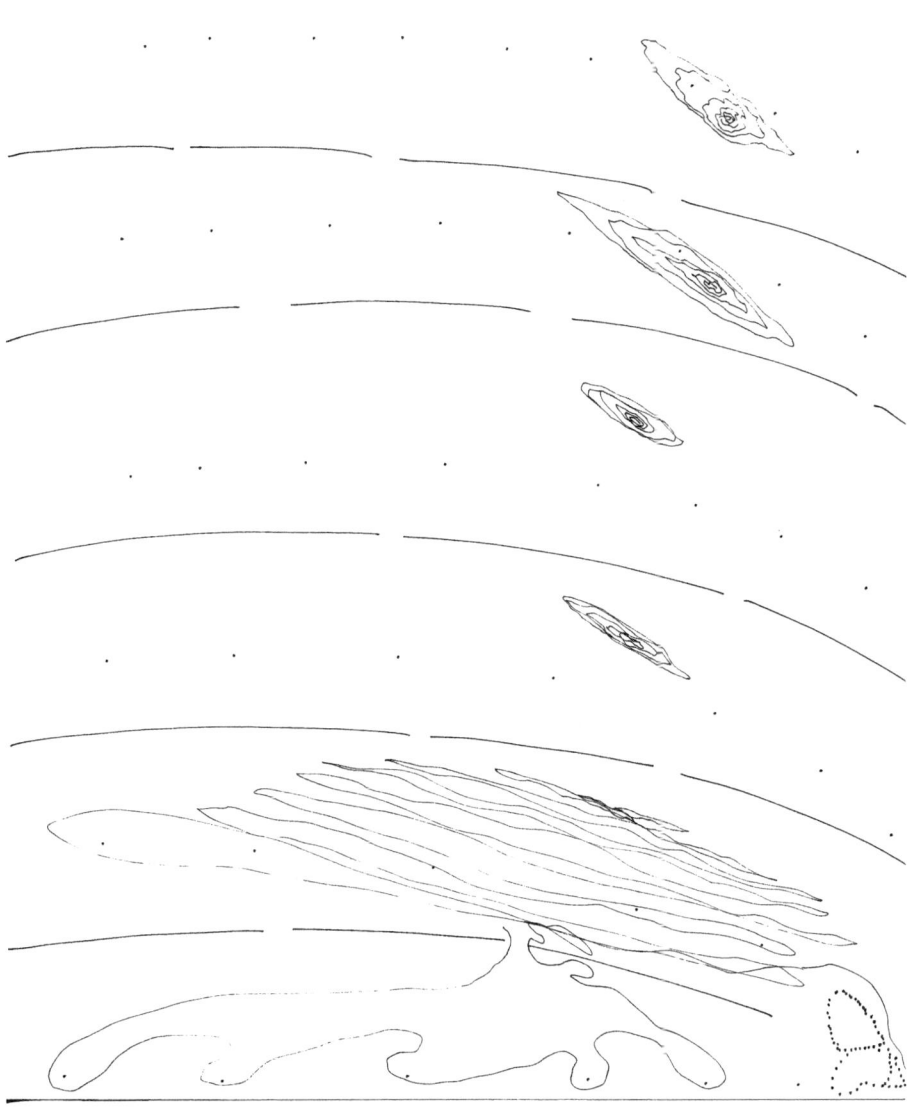

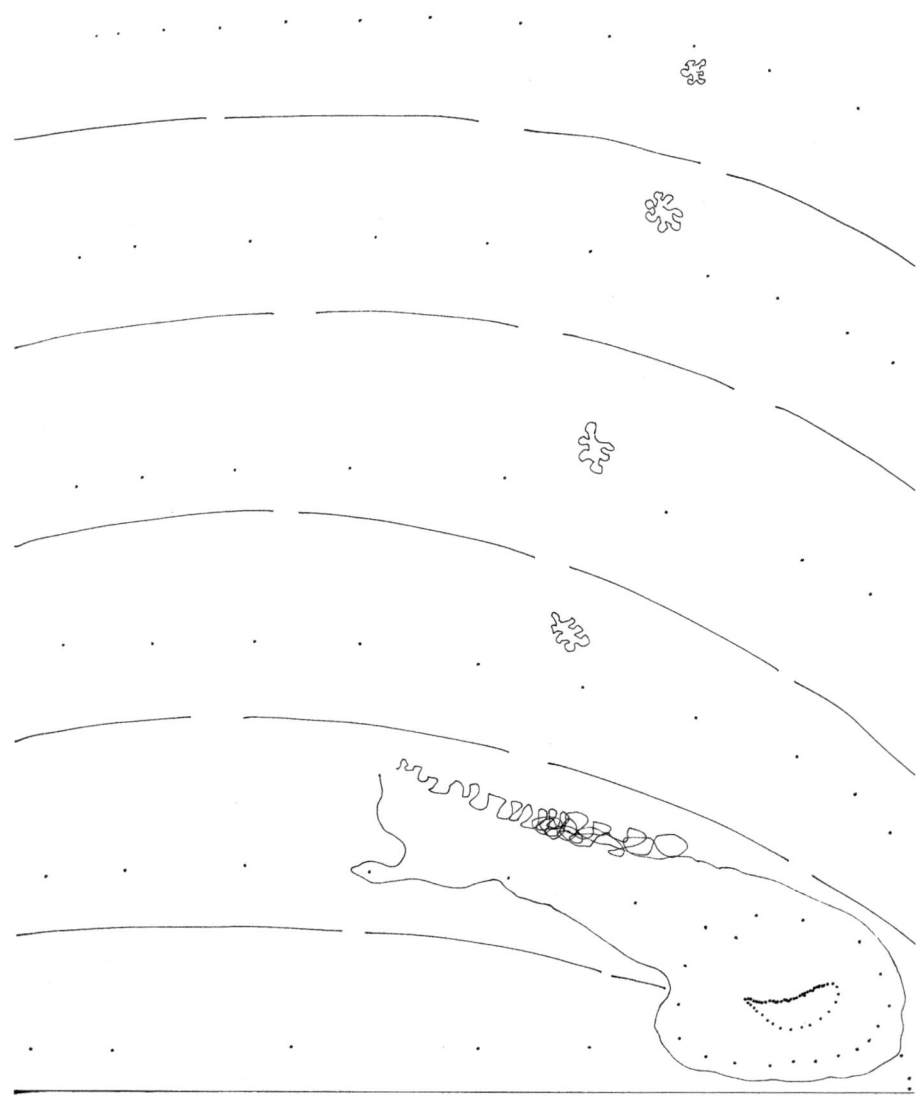

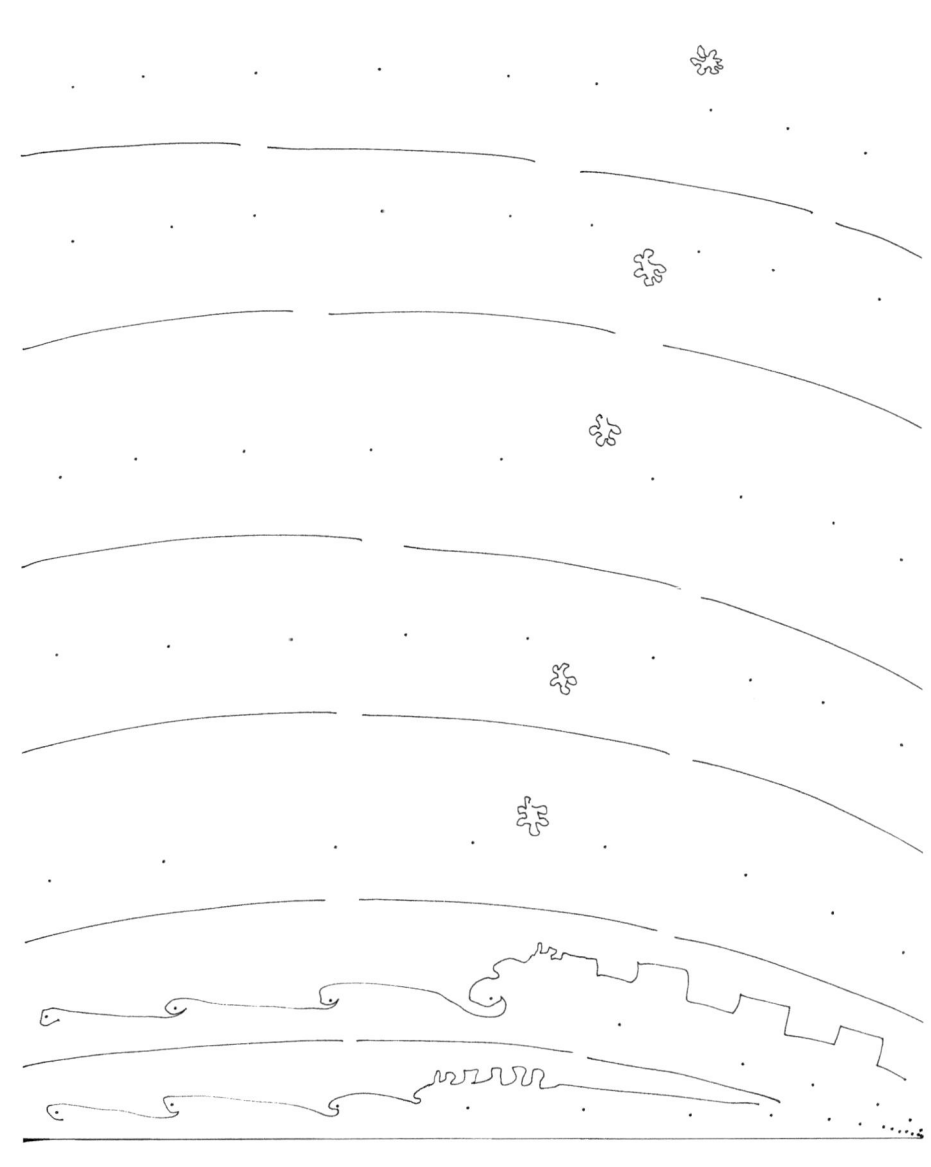

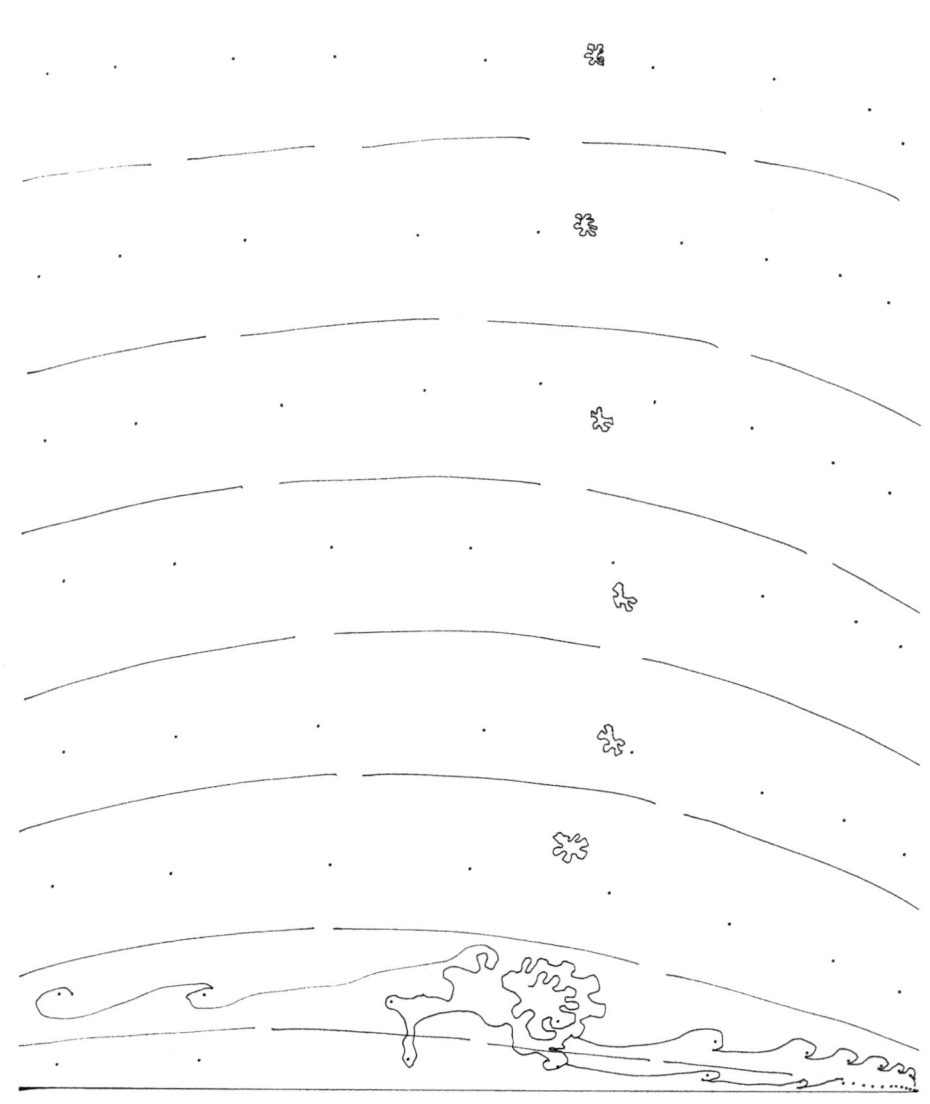

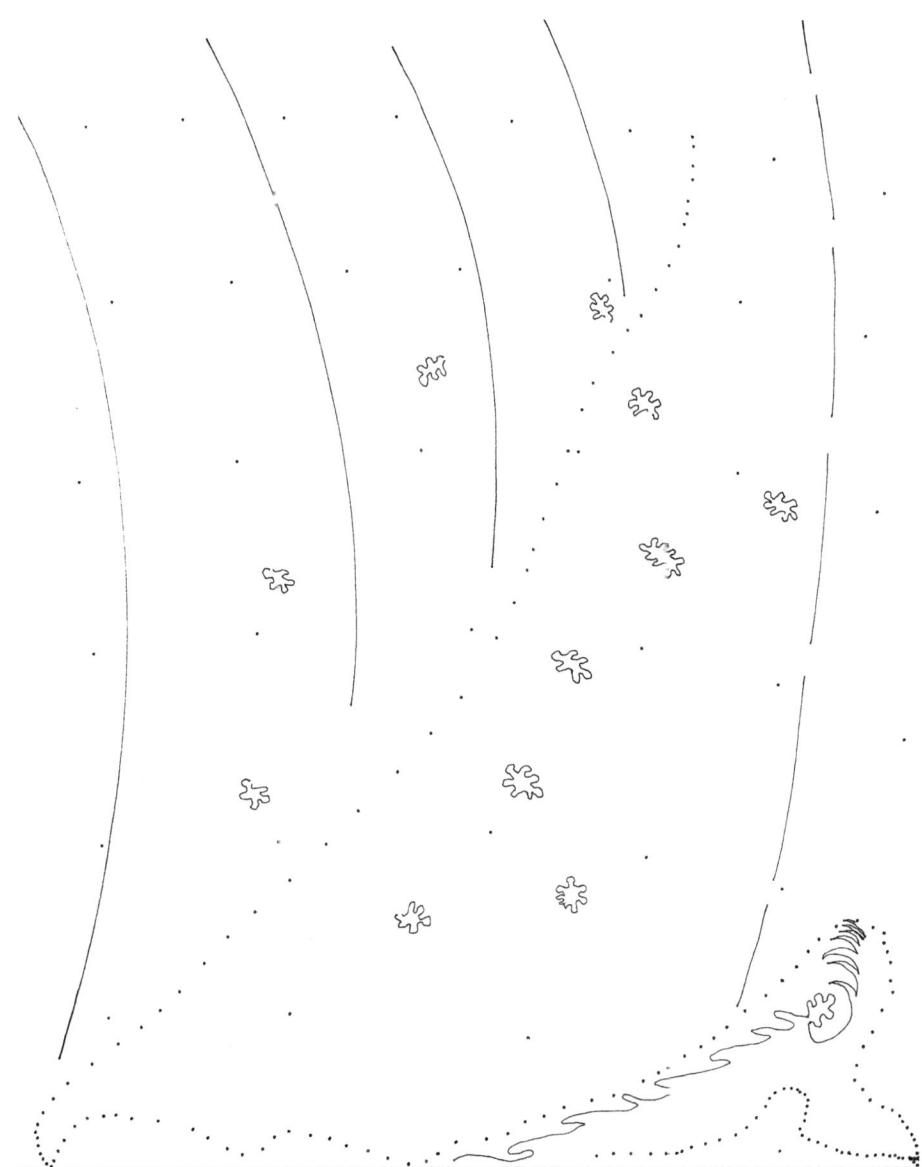

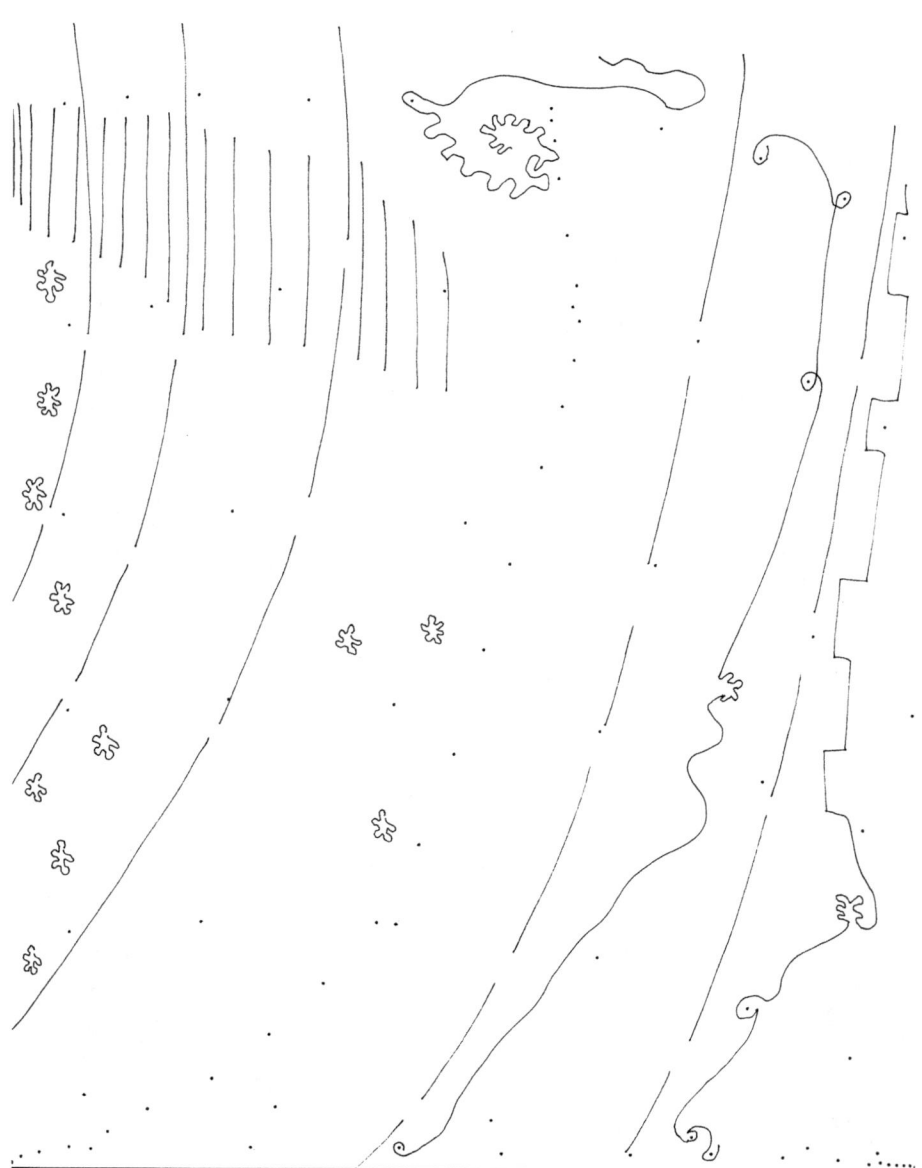

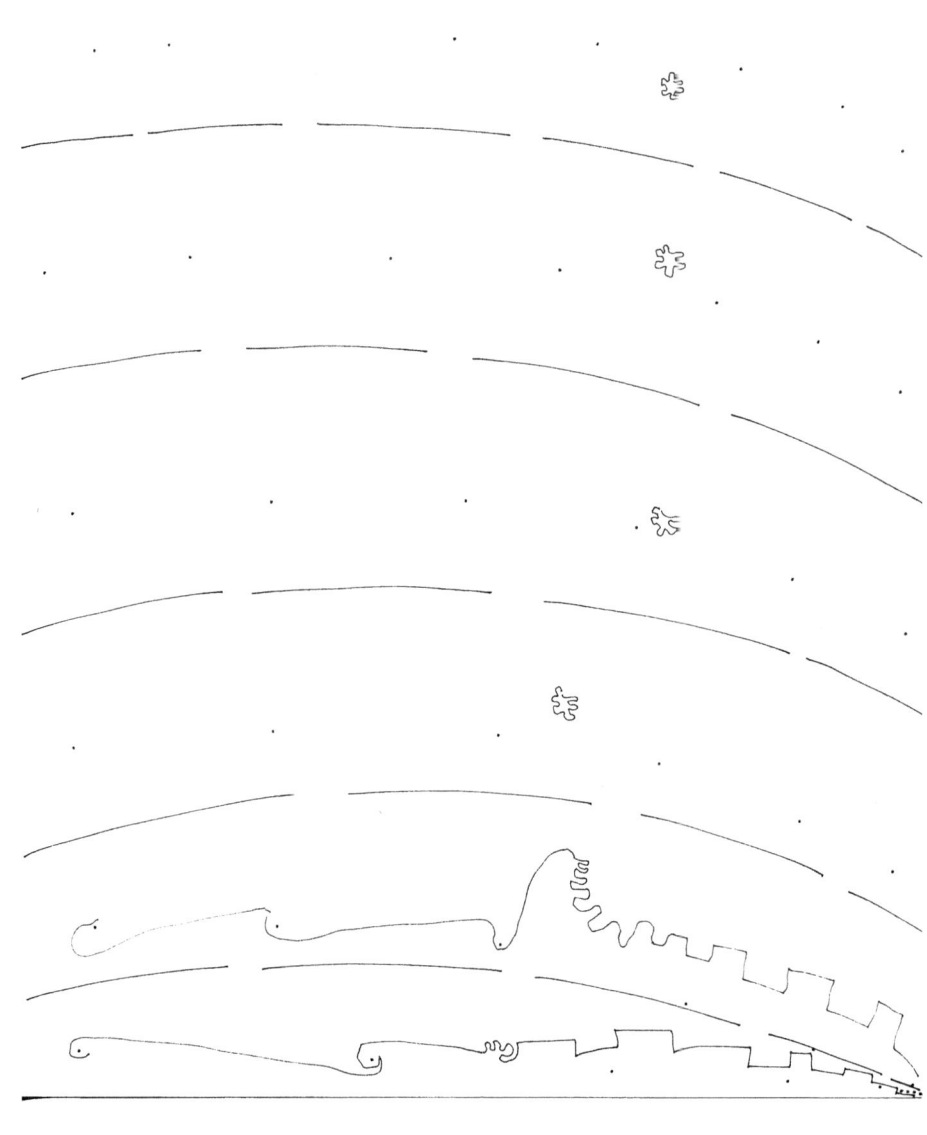

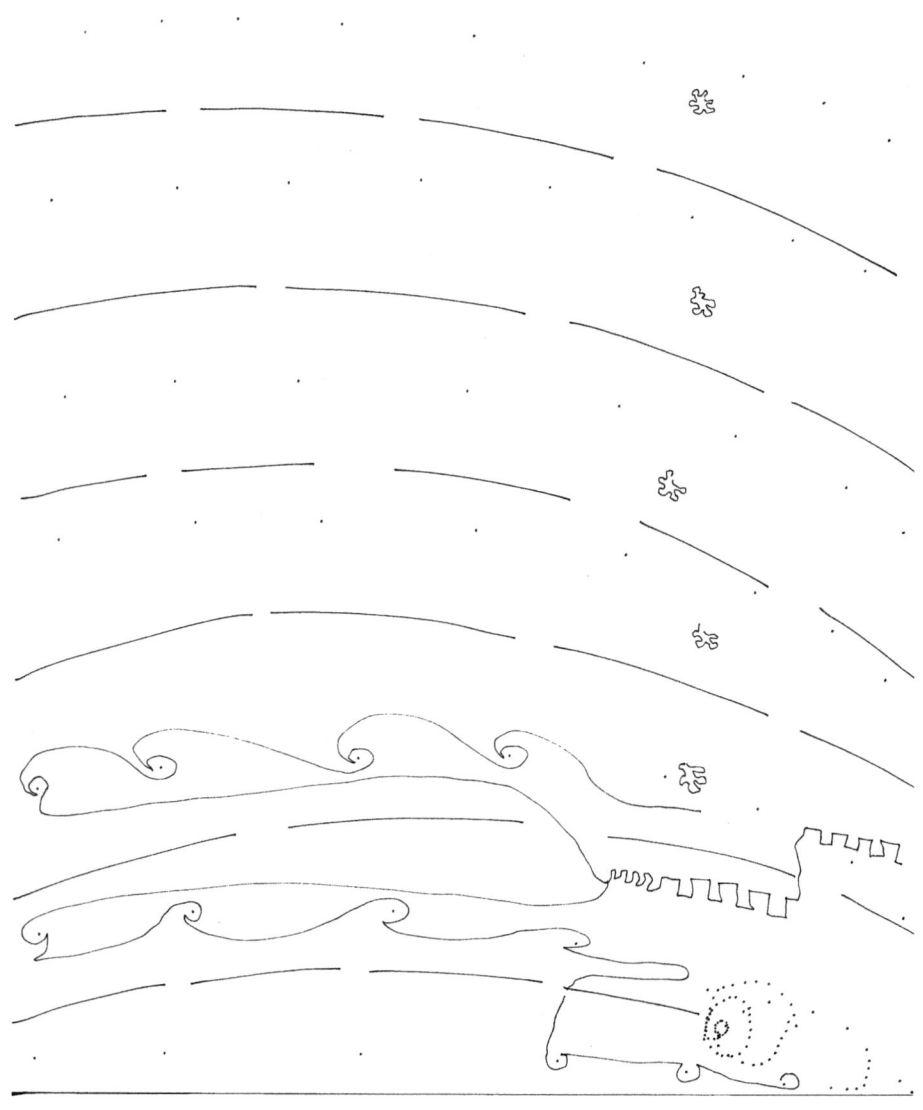

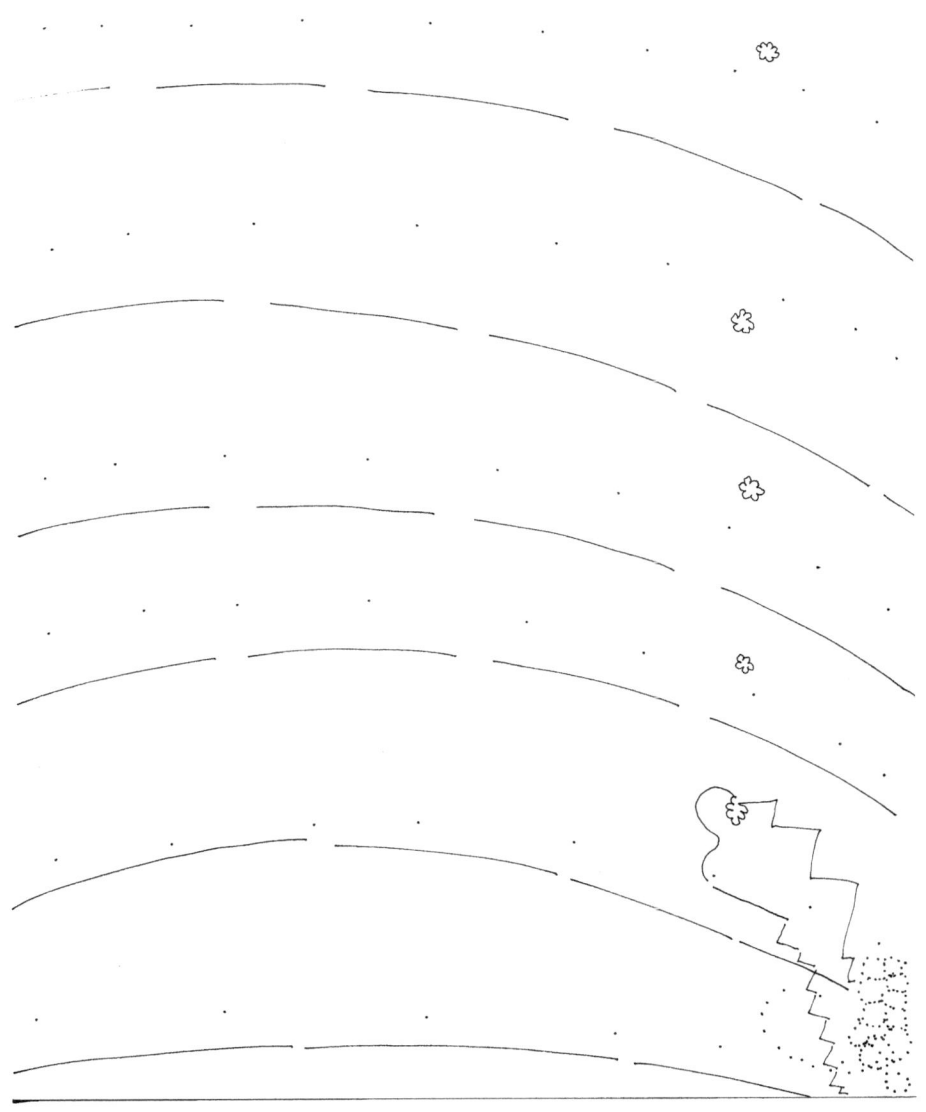

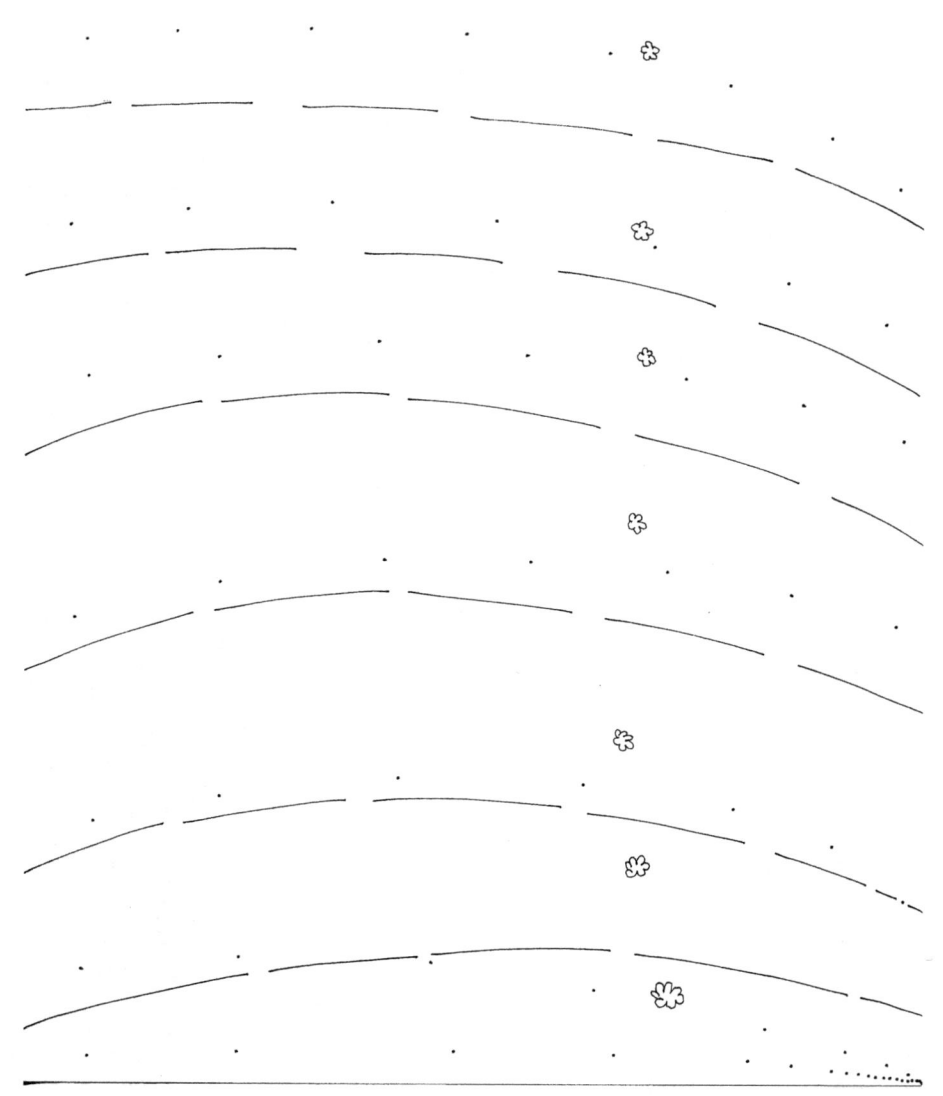

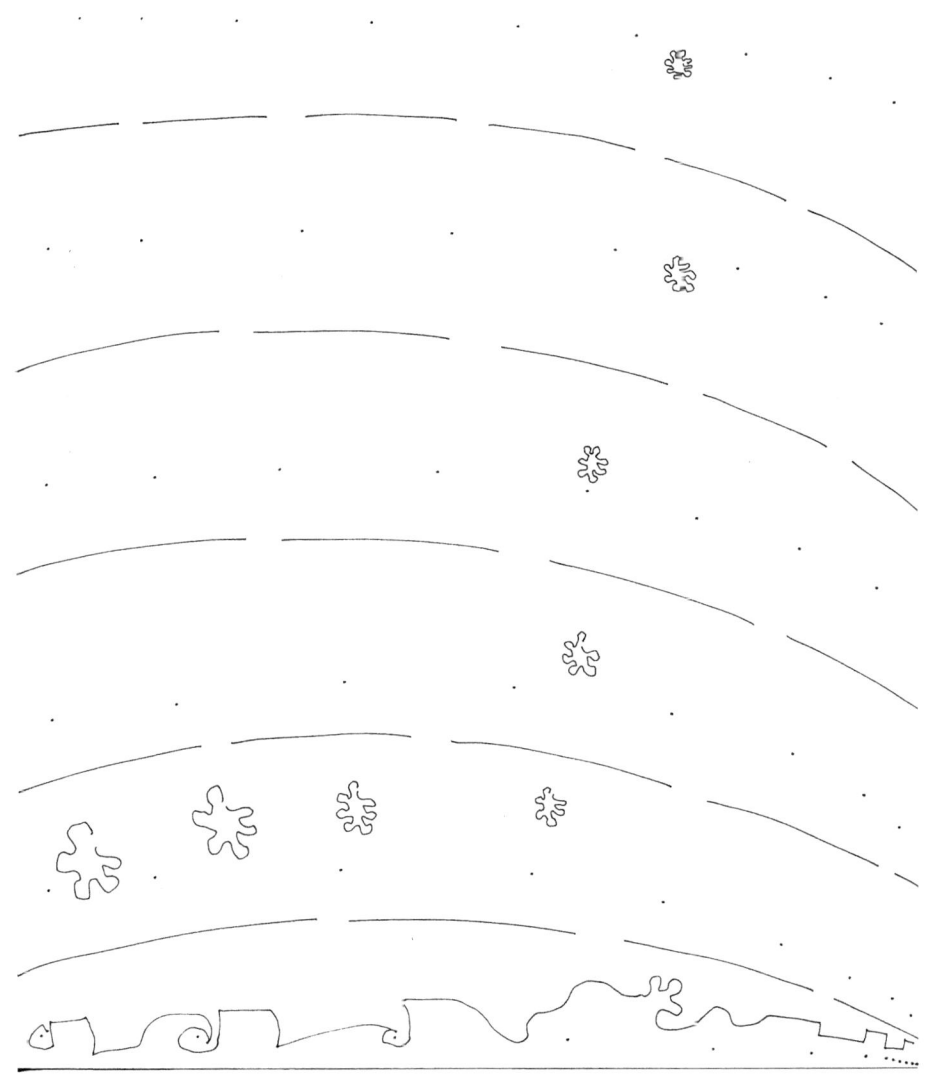

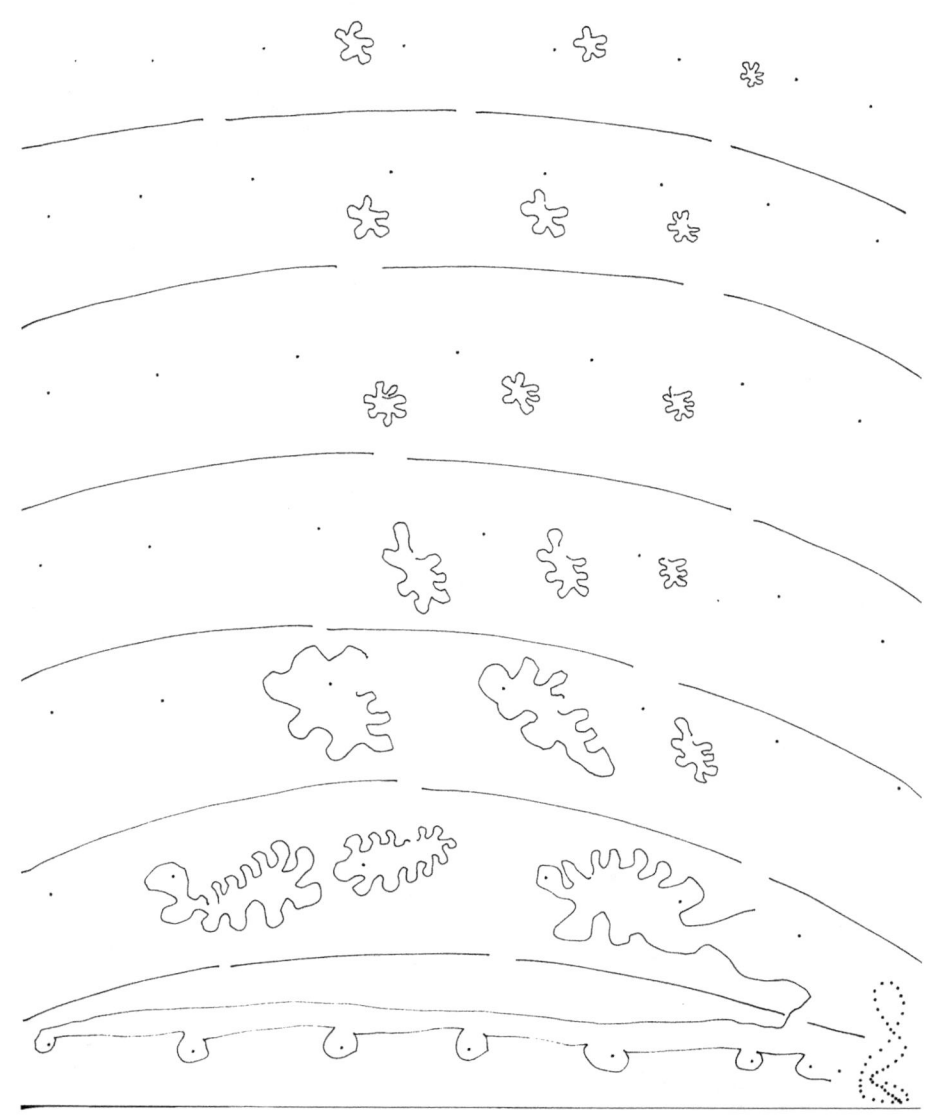

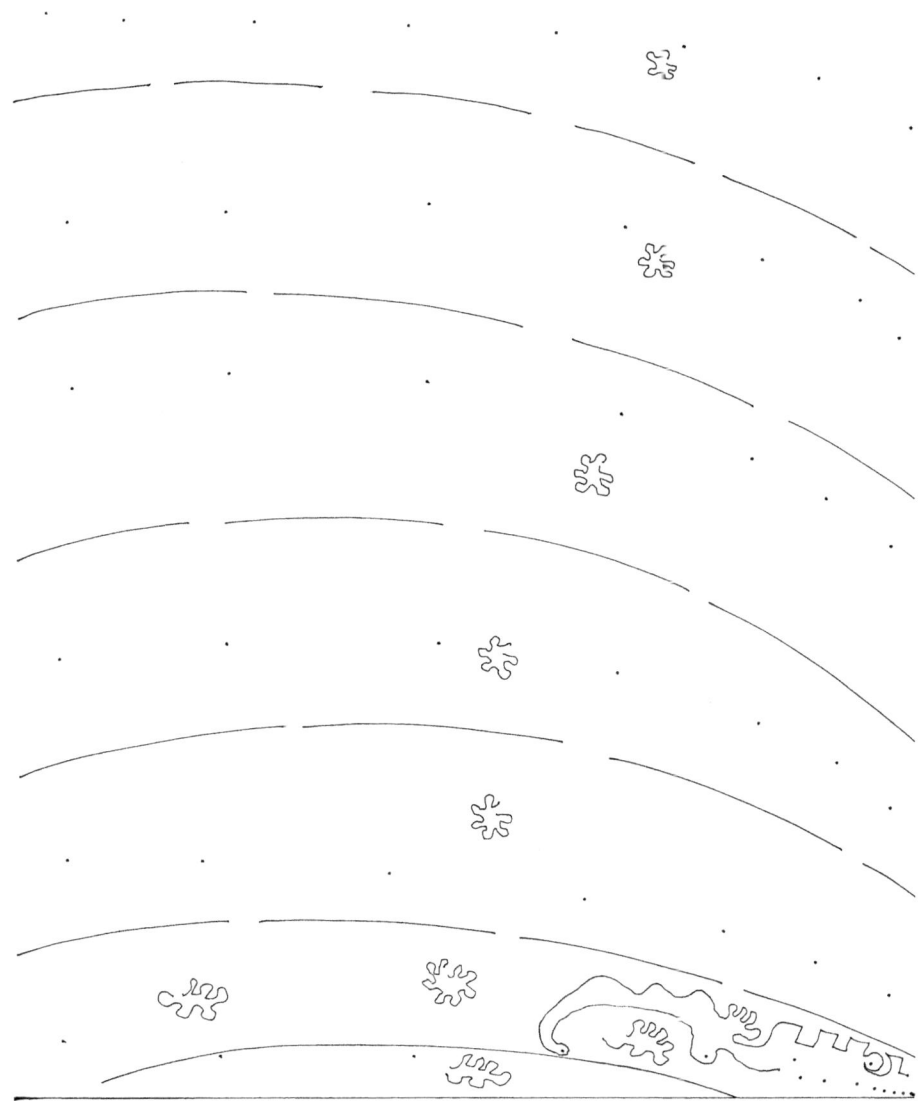

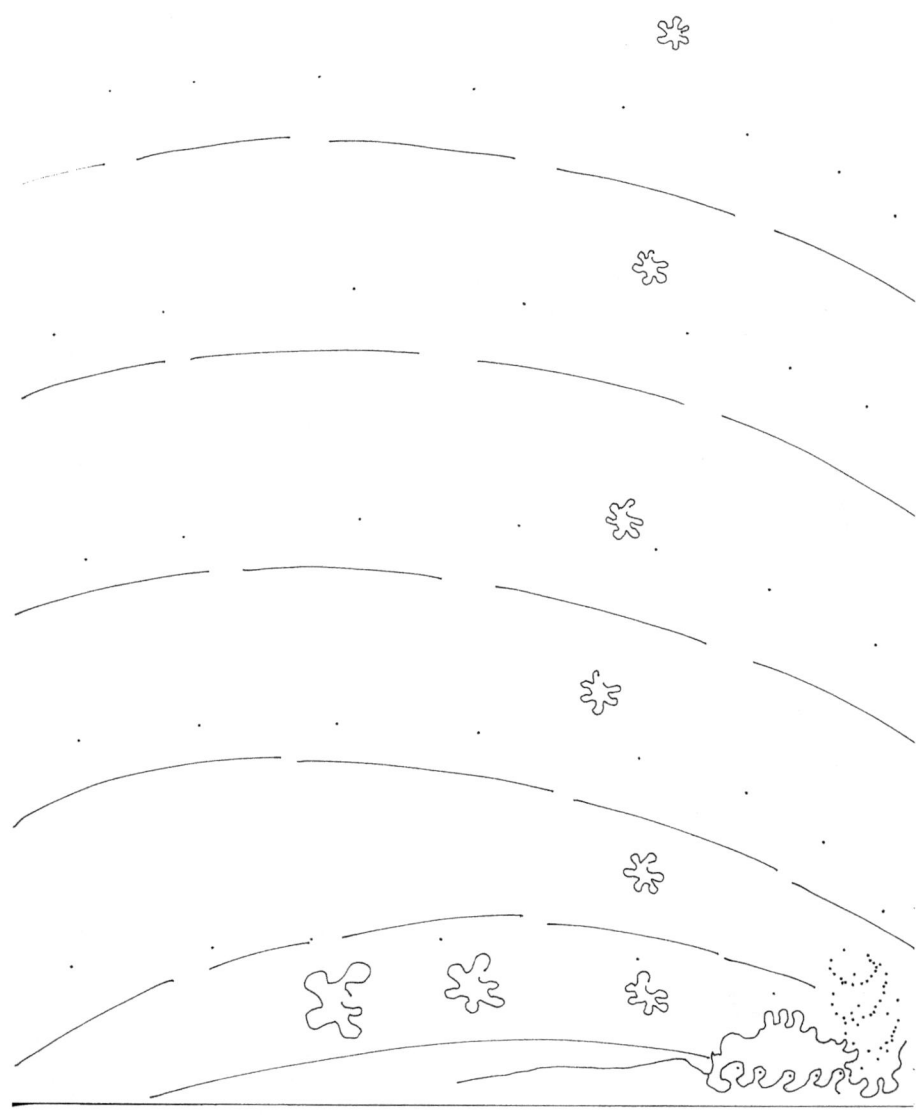

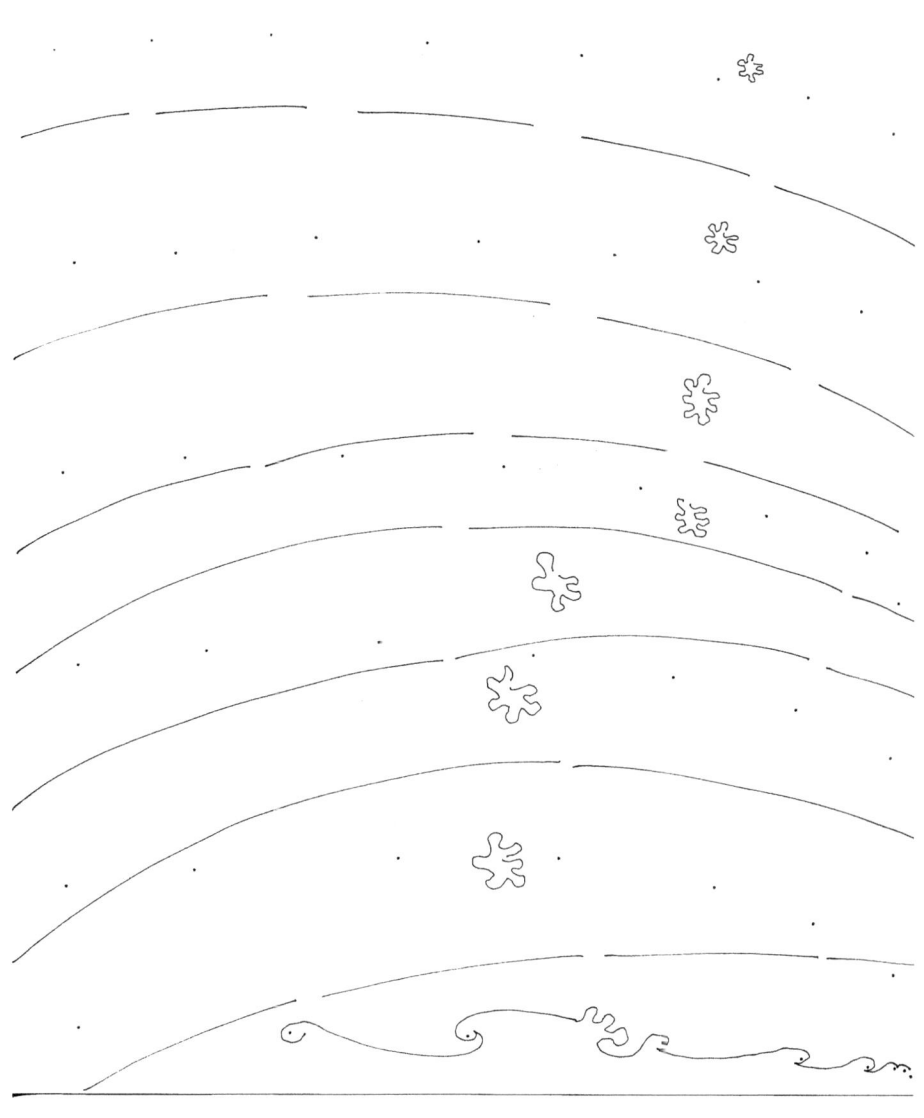

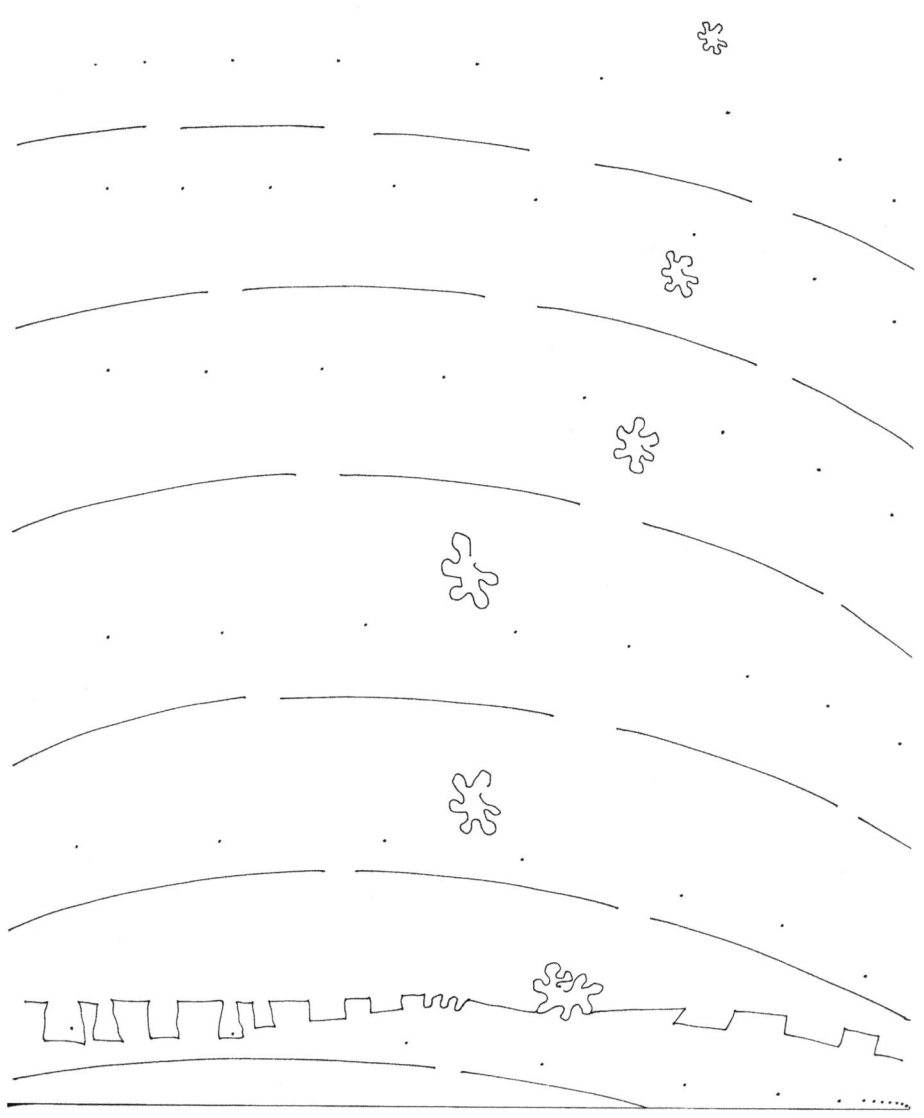

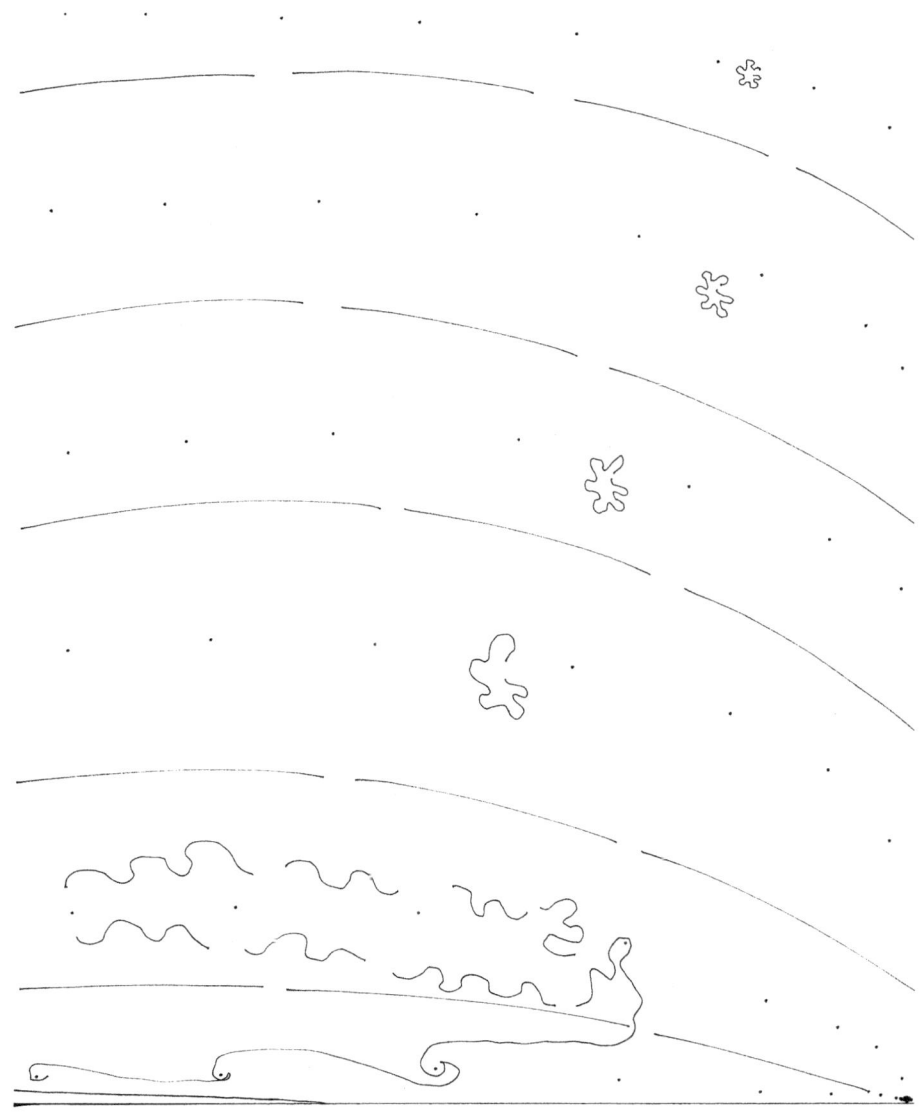

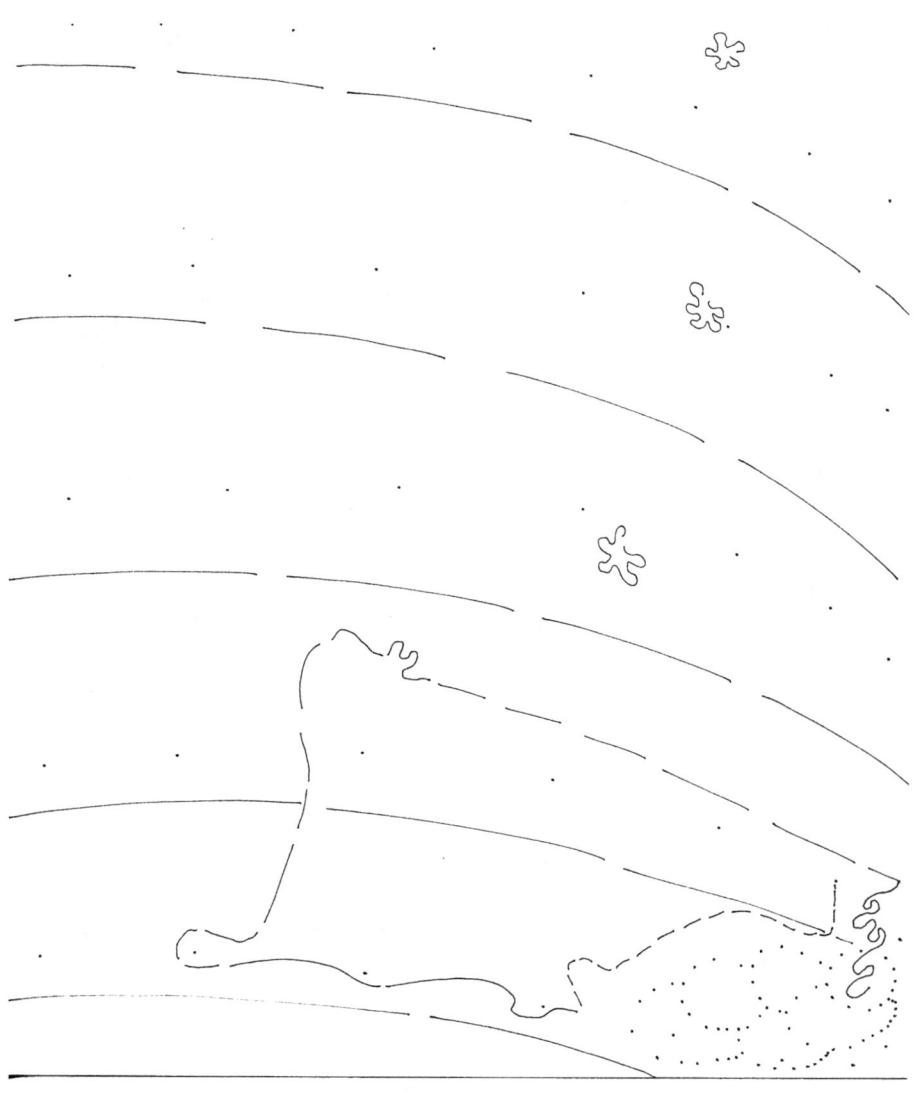

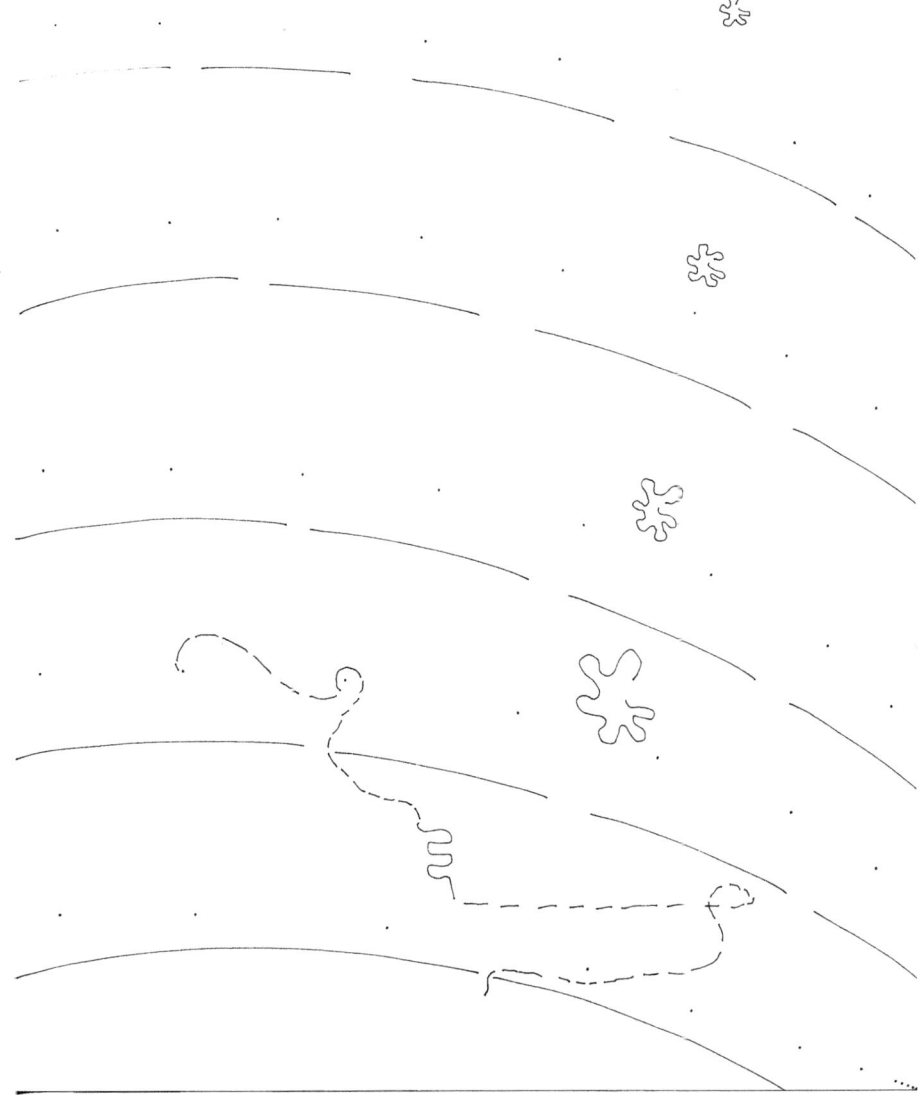

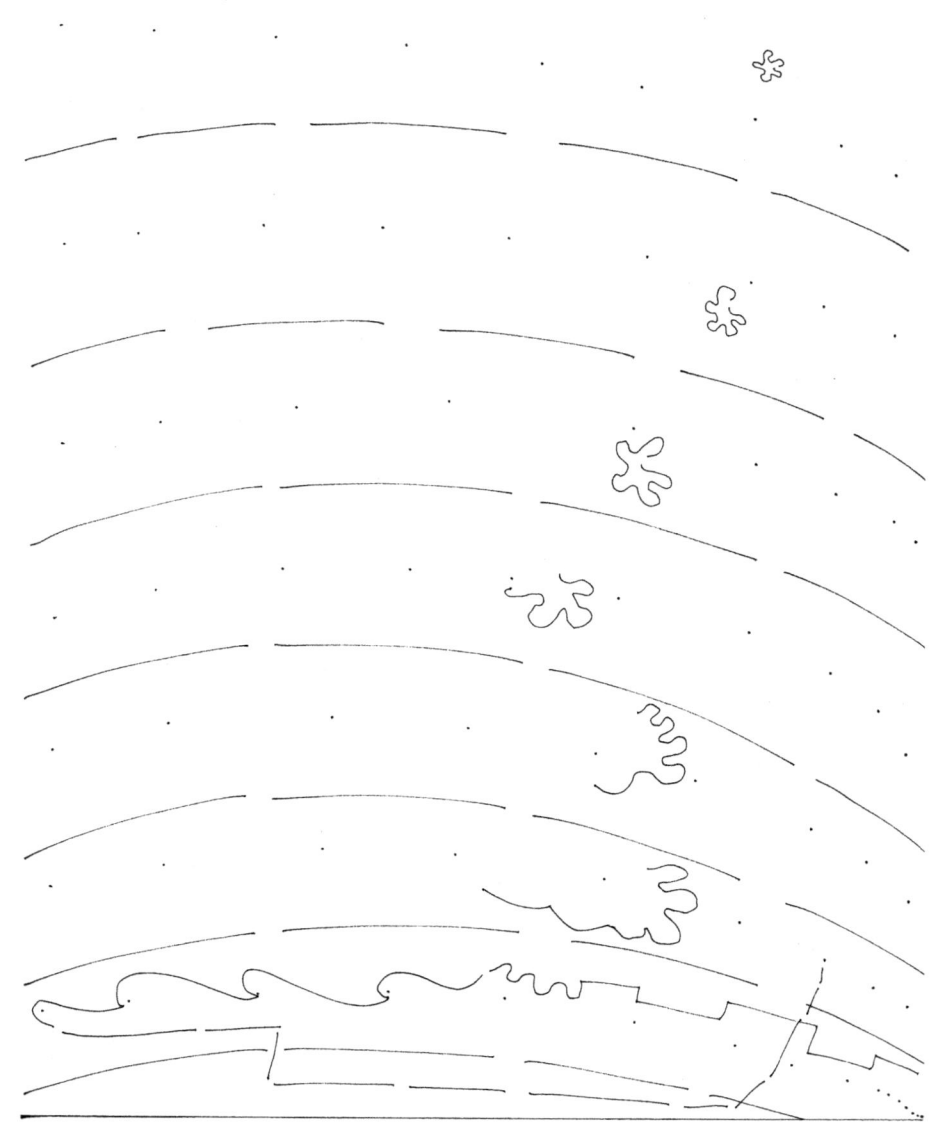

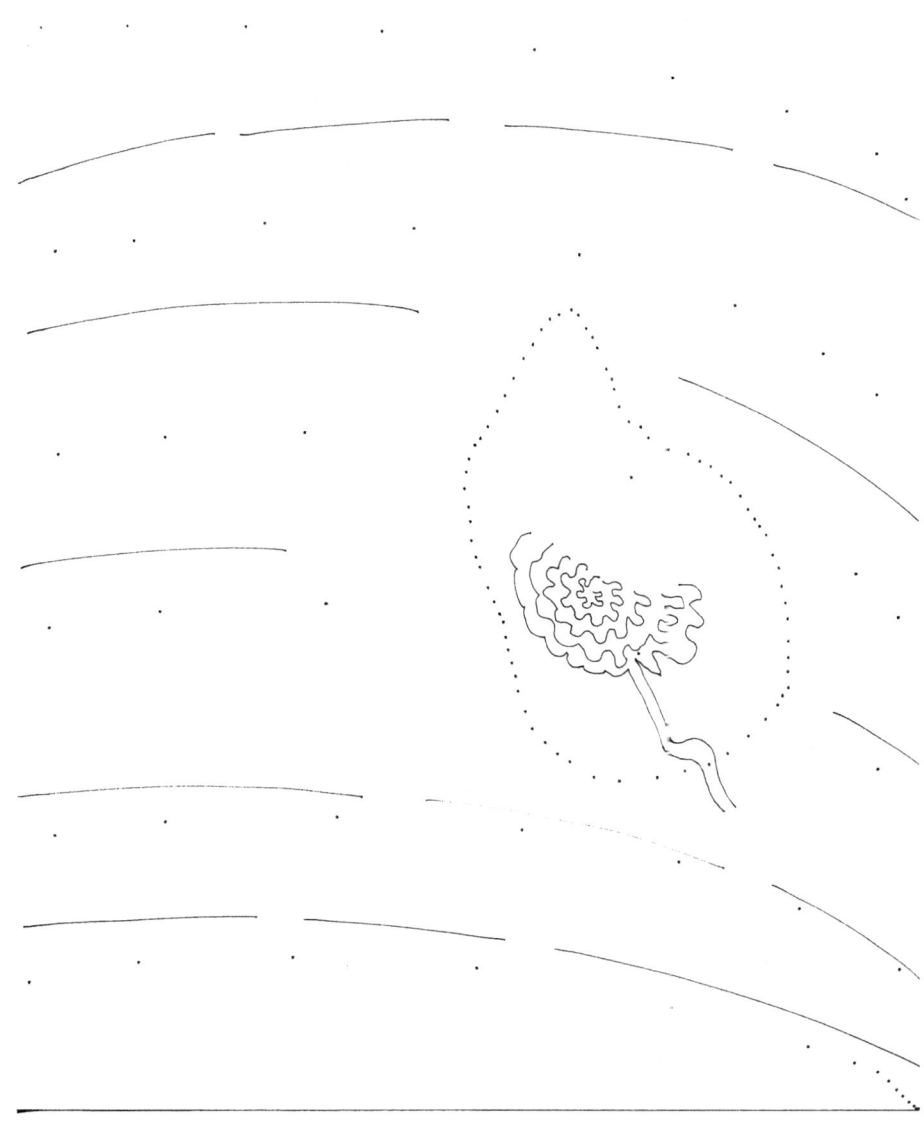

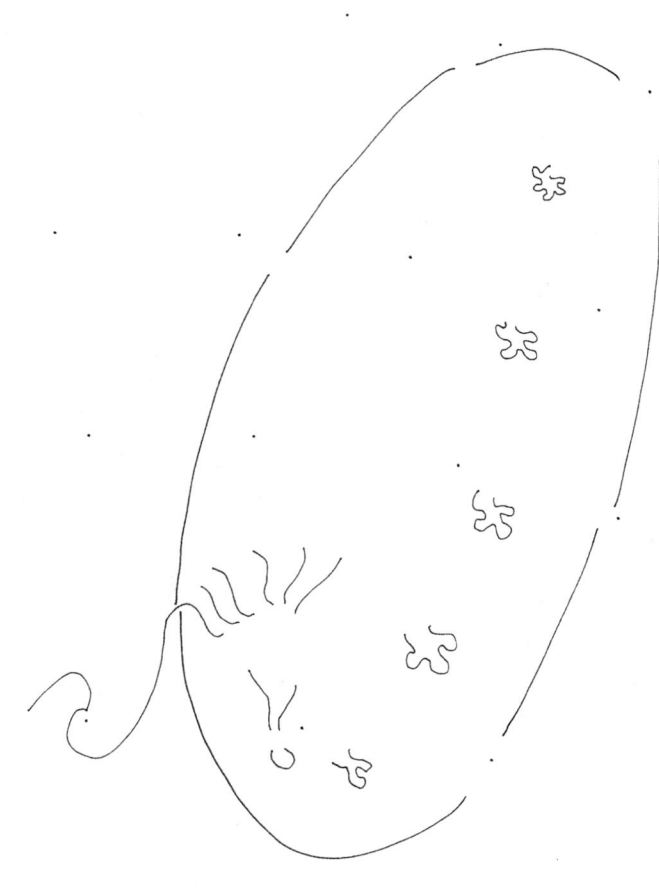

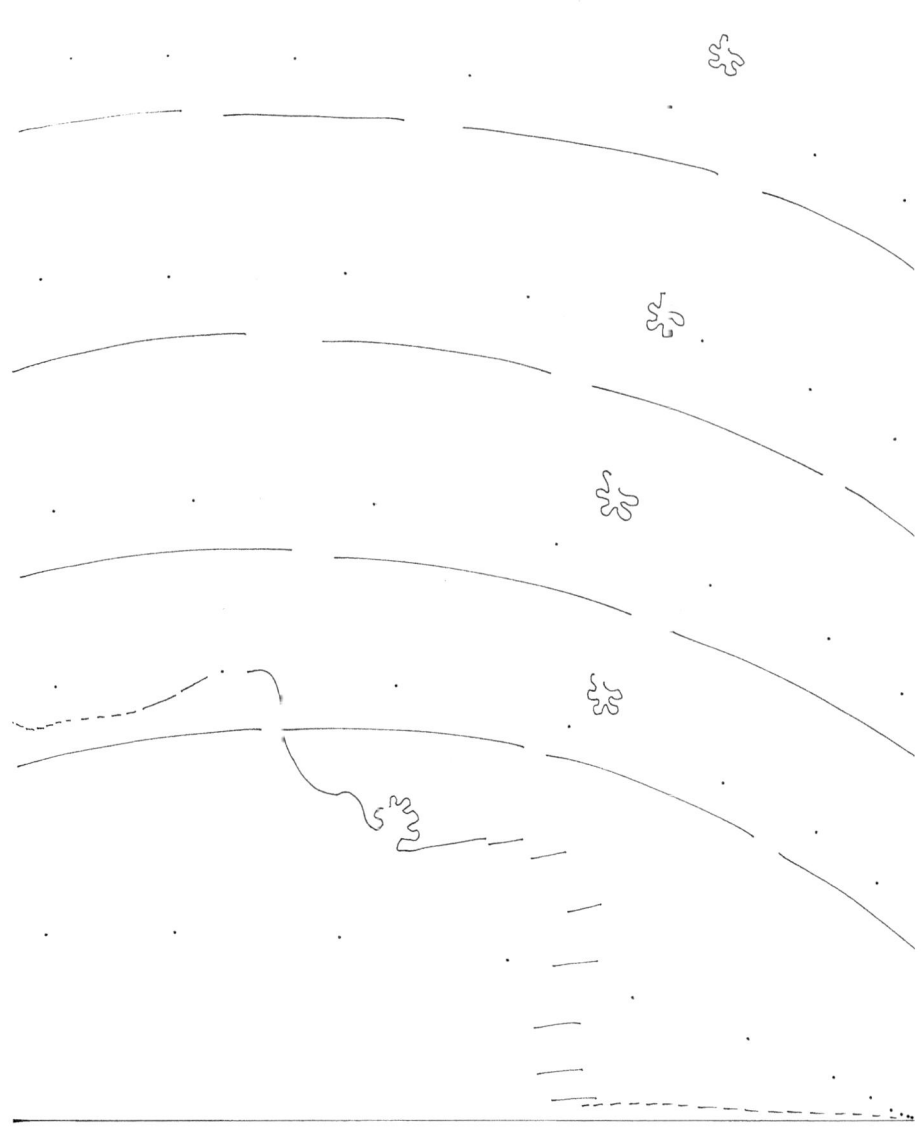

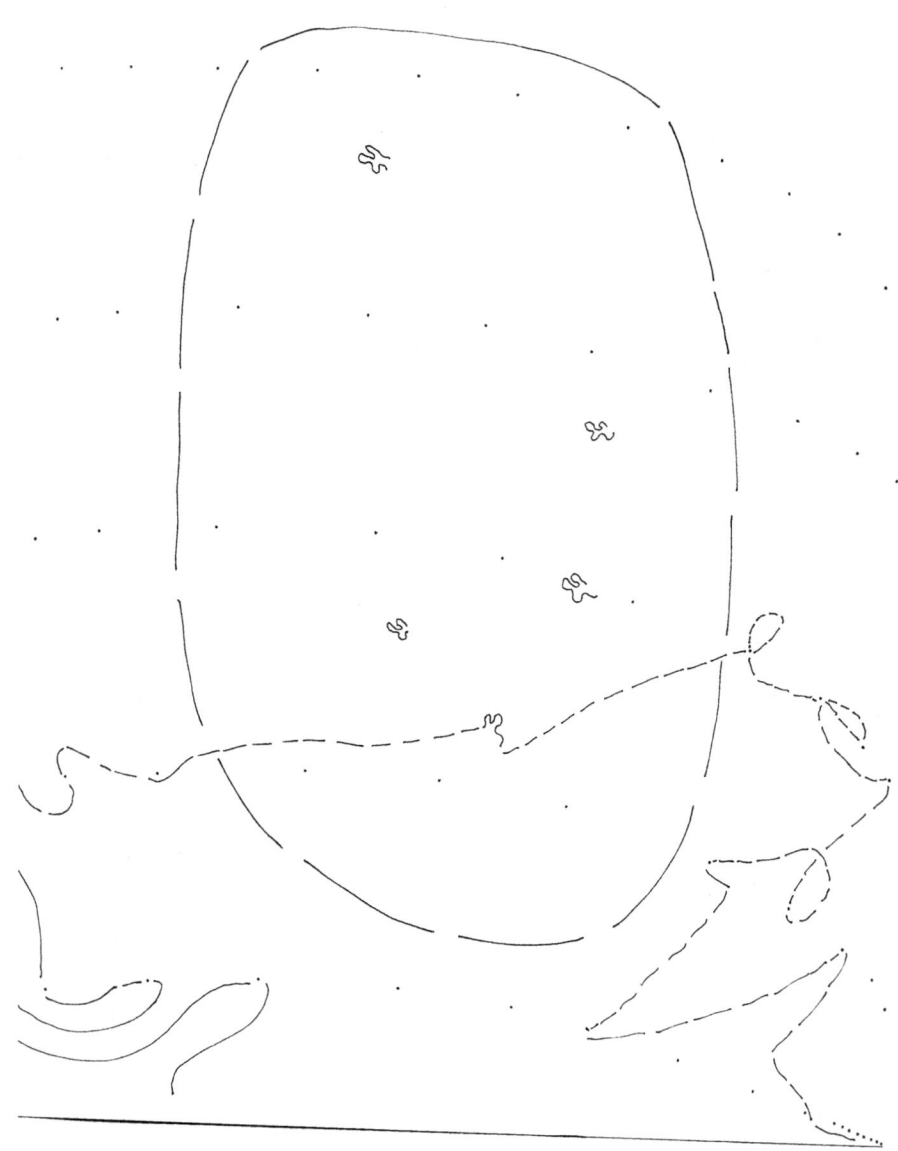

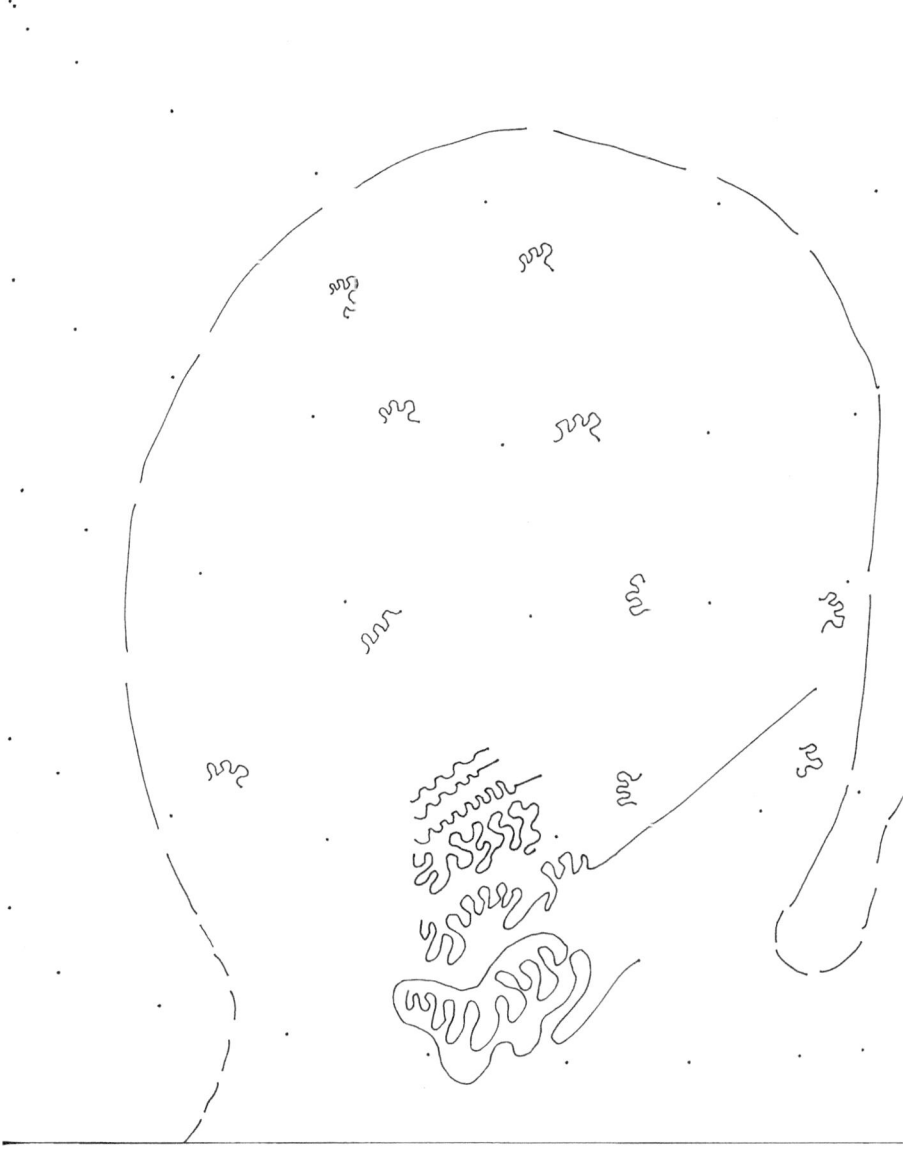

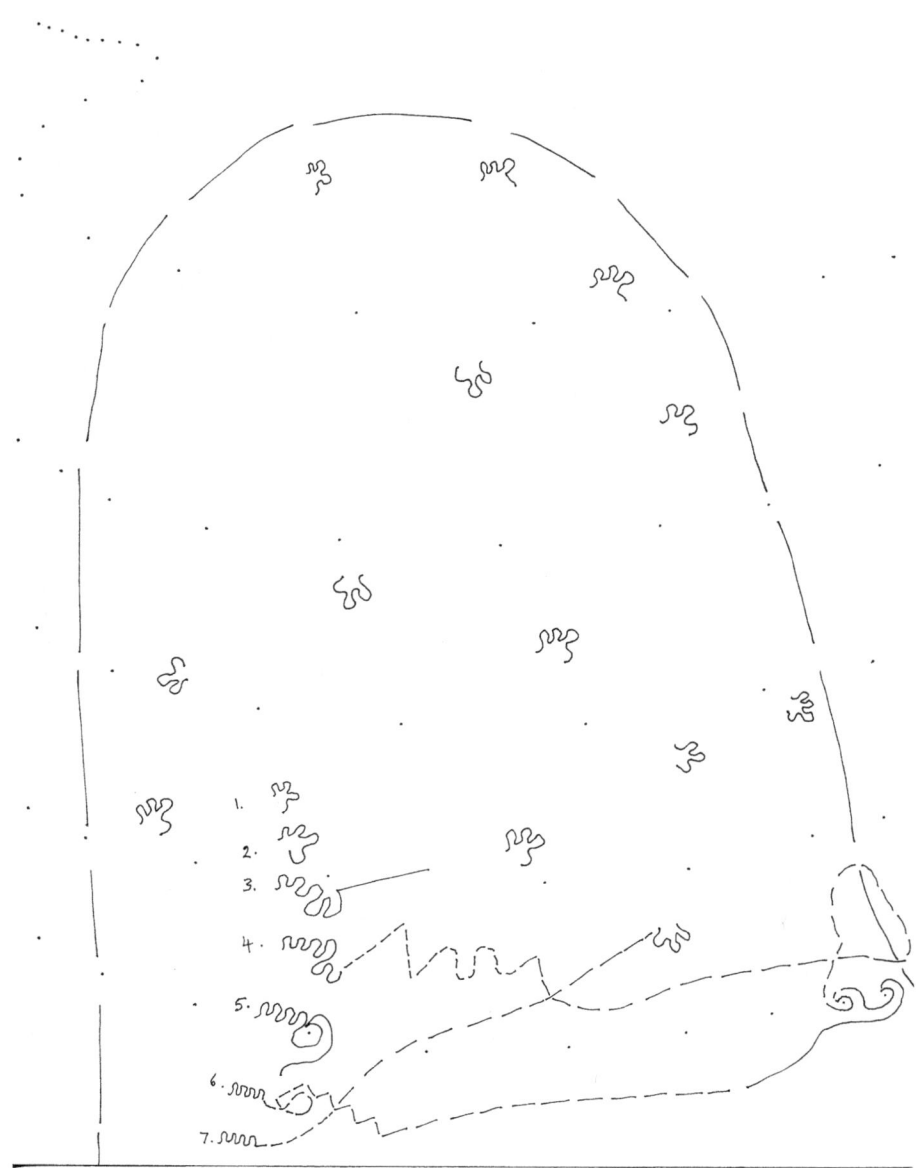

CONTINUED IN

VOLUME 3